TAKE
OFF
YOUR
GLASSES
AND
SEE

TAKE
OFF
YOUR
GLASSES
AND
SEE

*A Mind/Body Approach
to Expanding Your Eyesight and Insight*

Jacob Liberman, O.D., Ph. D.

*Three Rivers Press
New York*

Published by Three Rivers Press, a division of Crown Publishers, Inc., 201 East 50th Street, New York, New York 10022. Member of the Crown Publishing Group.

Originally published in hardcover by Crown Publishers, Inc., in 1995.

Random House, Inc. New York, Toronto, London, Sydney, Auckland http://www.randomhouse.com/

THREE RIVERS PRESS and colophon are trademarks of Crown Publishers, Inc.

Printed in the United States of America

Book and cover design by Laurie Zuckerman

Library of Congress Cataloging-in-Publication Data
Liberman, Jacob, 1947–.
Take off your glasses and see: a mind / body approach to expanding your eyesight and insight / by Jacob Liberman
1. Behavioral optometry. I. Title.
RE960.L53   1995   617.7—dc20   94–32101

ISBN 0-517-88604-9

10 9 8

This book is dedicated to the child within all

of us who has always been able to see.

It is only with the heart that one can see rightly; what is essential is invisible to the eye.

—Antoine de Saint-Exupéry,
The Little Prince

Contents

CONTENTS

List of Illustrations

Acknowledgments

Special Acknowledgment

I'd like to offer an especially heartfelt acknowledgment and thank-you to Rose Brandt for her friendship and loving support throughout the writing of this book.

Her exquisite personal sensitivity, combined with her skill as a writer, allowed her to transform my spontaneously expressed feelings and ideas into the content of this book.

As a person who has transformed her own vision, Rose's ideas, experiences, and suggestions are sprinkled throughout the text. Her friendship and contributions to this project have been invaluable to me.

Acknowledgments

This book is a compilation of many personal experiences that over the last twenty years have been inspired and nurtured by the influence of many close friends and respected colleagues.

I wish to deeply acknowledge my colleagues Ray Gottlieb, Robert Michael Kaplan, Elliott Forrest, Bruce Rosenfeld, Larry Jebrock, Sam Berne, Marc Grossman, Amorita Treganza, Robert Pepper, Simon Grbevski, and Peter Fairbanks for their loving support. I'd also like to acknowledge the courage and pioneering insights of Larry Dossey, Bernie Siegel, and Deepak Chopra.

I'd also like to thank my wonderful friends for their support and guidance over the years: Sky and Rainbow Canyon, Herb Ross, Paul and Grace Durga Lowe, Rose Kahn, Buzzy and Gayle Gordon Kaufman, Ron Henry, Terry and Suzanne Levy, Elio Penso, Richard and Marilyn Fendelman, Truth Paradise, Paul and Myra Berger, Stephen Feig, Eva and Herb Finkel, Frank Levinson, Maxine Rose, Alan Lauer, Laura Lea Cannon, Stephen Rose, Patricia Bell, Fred Spanjaard, Tom and Patricia Overton, Michael Greenburg, Brendan and Terry Hart Roberts, Bija Bennett, and Gerry Sindell. I'm very grateful to Suzy Hailperin and Cheryl Lynn Russell for their support during my early years of discovery.

To my loving parents, Joseph and Sonia Liberman, and my exquisite children, Gina and Erik Liberman, I'd like to express my deep love and appreciation.

I also wish to thank my agent, Loretta Barrett, my editors Erica Marcus and David Groff, and Crown Publishers, for believing in me, giving me the opportunity to share my vision, and guiding me to its completion.

Foreword

This book, which Jacob Liberman originally entitled *Seeing,* is much more than advice by a former optometrist concerning eyesight. It is a deeply transformational approach to the broader subject of vision.

We understand vision, metaphorically, as perception that extends beyond the currently given. "Visionary" artists, for example, are those who give us "visions" of a future that are more than extrapolations from the present. A person of "vision" is one who sees what is coming and prepares for it appropriately.

In physical terms, "vision" means "eyesight." These two understandings are now merging into a more comprehensive and expanded experience of vision.

The human species is undergoing an unprecedented transition. The experience of what it means to be a human being is changing. Among these changes is the expansion of human perception beyond the limitations of the five senses. As more and more humans begin to gather and utilize data that the five senses cannot provide, the definition of "vision" is expanding beyond the capability of the eyes to see physical objects.

For example, when a mother "sees" that her daughter, returning to college, has driven off the road and rises in alarm at the moment that the car begins to roll toward trees, she is experiencing a "vision" that does not originate in her physical eyes.

When a man on an operating table, deeply anesthetized, "sees" the procedures that his surgeons and nurses are performing on him, and the color of the socks that they are wearing, he is using a "vision" that is not limited to what his eyes can detect.

This book is about the expanded experience of "vision." It is a reflection of and a product of the evolutionary transition that is under way. Jacob Liberman has begun the process of expanding his former discipline—in this case, optometry—to encompass the expanded reality of multisensory humans, humans who are not limited in their perception to the five senses.

This same process of expansion is occurring in every aspect of human experience. It is especially noticeable in the sciences, which, until recently, drew their strength from rigorous exclusion of all that is not detectable by the five senses, that is, all that cannot be empirically verified.

Health, for example, is now recognized to be more than physical, and physical health is now acknowledged to have nonphysical roots. The relationship of stress—emotional toxins—to physical health is becoming as evident as the relationship of physical toxins to physical health.

The purpose of this book is to establish the larger context of vision in which eyesight occurs. It is of value to every individual whose awareness of himself or herself is expanding beyond identification with his or her physical capabilities, and not only to those who wear glasses.

It is the natural development of a discipline that concerns itself with vision. It establishes in the terms of this discipline the same expansion beyond physical circumstances that will soon characterize every human activity.

The ideas that Jacob Liberman shares improve not only vision, but also eyesight. It is this aspect of the book that has inspired its title. I wore glasses from grade school until reading this book. I do not wear them now, except to drive, even though I previously experienced headaches, which I associated with "eye strain," whenever I took them off for more than half an hour. The unaided visual acuity of both of my eyes combined improved from 20/70 to 20/60—one line on the eye chart—merely by following Jacob Liberman's advice: "Close your eyes, inhale. Exhale, softly, and open your eyes gently. Do not look at the chart. Let the chart look at you. Don't try to grab a line with your mind. Look at one letter, and let it come into focus."

Letters on the 20/50 line now come briefly into focus—the same experience that preceded my ability to read the 20/60 line. This is considered impossible by most optometrists and ophthalmologists.

More than all else, this book is about awareness and a state of being that Jacob Liberman calls "effortless learning" and "effortless living." He demonstrates, in terms of physical eyesight, that "the harder you try, the less you see," and expands that experience beyond visual acuity. It is here, at the heart of what Jacob Liberman shares, that the book has nothing to do with glasses and eyesight. The "exercises," actually engaging games, that he provides tap an intelligence that the intellect cannot access.

I first experienced effortless learning as a student at Harvard. My small-town education did not prepare me for Harvard. I was a mediocre student there. I applied myself hard, but barely managed to get Bs.

One assignment was to compare Freud's *Totem and Taboo* with Emile Durkheim's *The Elementary Forms of the Religious Life,* a thick volume of small print and closely spaced lines, all mind numbing to me. To *read* Durkheim's work would have taken me a month, provided I had nothing else to do. I put the paper off and off and off until it was due the next day.

When I sat down at the typewriter, I had no time to even attempt to read these books. I skimmed through Freud's book, literally thumbing through the pages, underlining anything interesting. Then I did the same with Durkheim's. I noticed that here and there some of Durkheim's ideas seemed either opposed to or in alignment with Freud's. I marked those places and then typed whatever came to me about the two. I had no choice. I *had* to hand in *something.*

That paper was the first and only A+ that I got at Harvard. It was interesting and fun to write. I was relaxed and rather enjoying myself while I wrote it—as much as I could knowing that I was going to get an F, or a D at best. It was beyond my comprehension that so little effort could produce such a stellar result. I thought that I had to struggle with my limited intellectual capability merely to pass my courses at Harvard, and I had become accustomed to feeling overwhelmed.

My next experience with effortless learning came about fifteen years later when I wrote *The Dancing Wu Li Masters: An Overview of the New Physics*. I had never written a book or studied physics, but I delighted in doing both for the first time, and the book won the American Book Award.

My experiences with effortless living began only recently, and to my great surprise and joy.

This book goes directly to the experiences of effortless learning and effortless living. They are intimately part of the vision that this book is designed to develop. They are goals that all desire—those who wear glasses, and those who do not. They result from changes in awareness, not optics, and thereby reflect the emerging understanding within the emerging humanity that awareness changes *all* experience without exception.

—Gary Zukav

Introduction
Seeing from the Heart

What is vision? How do we see? Do our eyes really work just like a camera lens? Do we even see with our eyes? Why do the eyes appear to be the only part of the physical body that is not self-healing? Why is the modern world experiencing an epidemic of vision problems? Why do eye-care specialists almost unanimously assume that preventive or remedial vision care is wishful thinking at best? Why do we continue to prescribe glasses for vision problems that only continue to deteriorate? Could wearing glasses actually contribute to the progression of poor vision? What is the relationship between our vision, our beliefs, and our emotional state?

I was just beginning to practice optometry twenty years ago when these questions began to weigh on my mind. I felt that I had to do *something* to find the answers. My solution was to begin an experiment on the workings of my vision. The startling result was a spontaneous healing—my eyesight instantaneously improved from almost 20/200 to better than 20/20. I knew that I had come upon something very important, because I had been taught that that kind of change was *impossible*. The only explanations that fit my experience completely contradicted everything I had learned in optometry school. So I left my training behind to develop a new approach to natural vision improvement, one that was based on the fundamental self-healing properties of the body/mind.

As I introduced this new approach to my patients, I noticed that it did a lot more than help people improve their eyesight. In fact, vision improvement was just a small part of the powerful transformations that began to occur. In the twenty years since then, I have seen over and over that changing your vision is the same as changing your life. Jonathan Swift said a long time ago that "vision is the art of seeing [the] invisible." My clinical experience has proven that he was absolutely right—clearing our vision allows us to, literally, see the parts of ourselves, of our lives, that were invisible to us before.

In the ancient traditions, the concept of "vision" did not refer to eyesight; it was synonymous with wisdom. Real wisdom, even what we call genius, flows naturally from the clarity of our perception. The belief that eyesight occurs only in our eyes limits more than our vision; it limits our entire worldview. The eyes have been described most accurately as the windows of the soul. Light energy enters our being through our eyes, but our vision of reality is determined more by what we see with our mind's eye than what we see with our physical eye. In fact, I've found that our eyesight is simply a reflection of our view of reality. So when the mind begins to see more clearly, the eyes also begin to see more clearly—and that shift can be instantaneous.

I now spend most of my time speaking and giving workshops all over the world, and everywhere I travel, I meet ordinary people who have miraculously healed their eyesight. They all suddenly *saw* a new possibility.

Vision is so much more than eyesight. The eyes are simply one focal point in a vast perceptive field. But if we live in a chronic state of fear or anger, all our sensory functions contract; we literally become narrow-minded. After a while that contraction begins to feel "normal." Most of us seem to have closed down some aspects of our perception. Even people with 20/20 eyesight may have very poor "vision." So whether you wear corrective lenses or not, this book can guide you to seeing more clearly and living more effortlessly, to creating your own spontaneous healing, your own miracle.

In our society, poor vision seems to have become a socially acceptable, even normal, substitute for self-awareness and emotional expression. This book will show how the suppression of feelings and perceptions has created the physical, psychological, and energetic roots of the current epidemic of vision problems. I'll also describe what I've found to be the most important aspect of vision improvement: the returning of our attention to those experiences that we have "blurred" out of our consciousness.

This book will explain how to begin that process, and it will also describe approaches that will support and complement that shift. We'll see how a deterioration of our vision results from the interaction of our thoughts, feelings, behavior, and social environment. We'll see how that process occurs as well as how to transform it with new habits that will support our ability to see clearly.

The first part of this book is devoted to expanding our understanding of vision and eyesight. Part Two describes practical techniques to improve eyesight—by relieving physical stress on the eyes and releasing emotional blockages. Part Three discusses how the way we see interacts with the way we think and learn, and presents a surprisingly fun, simple, and effective approach to the recalibration of the entire mind/body system for clear vision and effortless learning.

In general, the more we expand our self-awareness, the more deeply we are transforming our vision. However, almost any combination of the approaches and techniques described in this book may work for you. So use this book as a step-by-step manual, as a resource book to dip into and out of, or simply as an inspirational story. The most important aspect of clearing your vision is simply the willingness to consider new ideas, to be willing to experiment and discover what works best for you.

The old definition of vision kept us viewing the world through a hole rather than as a whole, but we are meant to see so much more. As Goethe said on his deathbed, "Open the second shutter, so that more light can come in." The real purpose of this book is to take you on a journey from seeing the world through a hole to seeing the invisible.

PART
ONE

There's More to Vision than
Meets the Eye

Before You Read Further . . .

YOU ARE about to embark on a remarkable journey into clearing your inner and outer vision. Since some people report vision improvement after simply being introduced to the idea, it's important to check the state of your eyesight before reading any further. This vision check does not replace a professional vision exam. It is just a quick way to get a rough baseline of your visual acuity at home. Just follow these steps (it's easiest to do this with a partner):

    1. Ask your partner to photocopy and assemble the eye chart on pages 111 to 114. Have him or her tape it to a wall at eye level, someplace where you can stand ten feet away from the chart. Don't look at the chart while the following steps are being done.
    2. Remove your corrective lenses—glasses or contact lenses.
    3. Measure off ten feet and turn to face the chart. Take a breath and relax. Beginning at the top with the largest letter, read all the letters out loud *without squinting or straining* (which may cause your vision to appear better or worse than usual). Your friend will stand near the chart to record

your accuracy, but should *not* give you any feedback until you are all done.

4. When you have read down as far as you can, have your partner read the tiny numbers on the side of the last line you read correctly. That is your baseline visual acuity. (If you've read down to the lines with many small letters, one or two errors per line are allowed if you've read the rest accurately.) If you can't read the largest letter on the chart, your baseline acuity is over 20/400. In that case, begin to approach the chart one foot at a time until you can read the first letter. Your baseline acuity is 20/400 at that distance: For instance, at eight feet, it is "20/400 at fifteen feet."

5. When you're done, cover the eye chart so you don't see it every time you walk by. If your friend would also like to check his or her vision, do it later or the next day, so that he or she has time to forget the letters that he or she saw on the chart.

As you begin to read this book, you will begin to look at your vision in a new way, and you may begin to notice some visual shifts. In the second section you will be asked to check your eyesight again and will be given further suggestions for using the chart to support the healing of your vision.

1 "Don't Worry, You'll Get Used to It!"

There is less in this than meets the eye.
—Tallulah Bankhead

HAVE YOU been told that you have progressive myopia (nearsightedness), hyperopia (farsightedness), astigmatism (visual asymmetry), or presbyopia ("old-age vision")? Have you been told that you will always have to wear glasses, at least for certain activities? Have you been told that the body has no natural way to reverse vision problems?

Most people have heard these statements at one time or another, and have believed them to be true—but are they? Have you ever wondered why our eyes—our most important sense, vision—are apparently the only organs in our miraculously self-regenerating body that lack the ability to correct their own imbalances? Why do doctors find it easier to believe a story of spontaneous remission of cancer than of self-correcting myopia?

Eye doctors tell us that 90 percent of us will need to wear glasses at some point in our lives. Another 70 percent of us, including many with 20/20 eyesight, unknowingly suffer from visual problems that are not even tested in the conventional eye examination.[1]

Yet my twenty years of clinical experience with vision care have repeatedly demonstrated that eyesight improvement is within the reach of virtually everyone. I've seen and heard of thousands of people who have improved their eyesight. It doesn't seem to matter how "bad" their vision is, how long they've had the problem, or what the problem is. The most significant factor in natural vision improvement seems to be in the mind, not in the eyes! Throughout this book, we'll be seeing that the way we think actually determines the way we see—and that something as simple as a shift in awareness is capable of instantaneously transforming our vision.

Over half the people in the United States wear corrective lenses, and almost all of them are capable of seeing much more clearly—if they would only experiment with changing their ideas about vision. As a practicing optometrist in the mid-1970s, I found that it came as quite a shock when I began to discover how our conventional beliefs about vision were keeping millions of us locked into limited eyesight and limited self-awareness! But I now realize that the conventional vision care that I was taught is designed not to treat (or heal) vision problems, but simply to mask the symptoms. Yet those symptoms are not just random—they are urgent signals that something in the body/mind is out of balance and *requires attention.* By sweeping those messages under the rug, conventional vision care may actually create more problems than it solves.

With a new way of seeing the world, I've been able to improve my own vision dramatically, and have helped thousands of others to reclaim their visual birthright.

"Don't Worry, You'll Get Used to It!"

By the time I graduated from optometry school, I had been wearing glasses for years, so I thought I knew all about vision care, both as a patient and as a doctor. It seemed pretty simple: My job as an optometrist was to help people see more clearly, right? But when I went into practice and began to work with people, things did not turn out the way I had expected.

At first, there wasn't that much to do—I didn't have anyone to practice on—but I was fortunate to be associated with a doctor who had a well-established office, so in the beginning I just watched him work. I quickly noticed that the practice of vision care seemed to follow a very repetitive pattern, which remained unchanged when I began seeing my own patients.

People of all ages would come into the office. Whether they were six years old or sixty, they would have the same complaint: "I can't see clearly." Children couldn't see the blackboard. Teenagers couldn't pass the driver's test. Middle-aged adults said their arms weren't long enough to read. Elderly people said their night vision was getting worse. The doctor's recommendations were almost always the same. If it was their first visit to the office, they would get a pair of glasses. If it was their second visit, they would get a second pair of glasses. If it was their fifth visit, they would get a fifth pair of glasses. Sometimes they asked for contact lenses instead of glasses. Sometimes they might get a few different prescriptions—distance glasses, reading glasses, bifocals, sunglasses, and so on. If they were fashion-conscious, they might buy several styles of eyeglass frames or colored contact lenses.

If it was a repeat visit, I would notice in reviewing their records that their basic complaint hadn't changed over time. The patients kept coming in with the same complaint, and I was trained to keep giving them the same solution. I couldn't understand it: If the problem kept getting worse, why did we keep using the same solution? It seemed very strange.

In school I had learned a comprehensive test procedure called the twenty-one-point examination. I would spend about an hour doing it with every patient. If you've ever had your vision checked, you know the routine. It takes you through a series of visual tests and such fascinating questions as "Which is better, number one or number two?" and "Tell me when these letters blur, break, and come back together again." I noticed that these questions often seemed to bewilder patients, as if they weren't sure they were answering them correctly. Sometimes they would ask to see the same pair of choices over and over again. Somehow we would come up with a set of answers, and I would compare the results to "the norm." (Every once in a while I'd wonder who had determined the prescribed norm on which every pair of glasses was based.)

People would usually leave the office feeling great. They had learned they didn't have cataracts or glaucoma or some strange eye disease, and a simple pair of glasses would renew the gift of sight. A week later they would return to the office to get their new glasses. As they put them on, they would suddenly stop in their tracks. "Yes," they'd say, "I can see much clearer now—but, gee, it *feels* very weird. My eyes *feel* like they're pulling. The room *feels* like it's distorted. The floor *feels* like it's tilting." Like every other eye doctor, I had been trained to respond, *"Don't worry, you'll get used to it."*

I couldn't understand that. The body was trying to tell us that something didn't feel right, and we just responded, *"Don't worry, you'll get used to it."* As I observed this happening to my patients, I remembered that every year I had received stronger and stronger glasses—and every year my eyes had continued to deteriorate. By 1973, I was wearing my eighth pair of glasses. I remembered the feelings of discomfort each time I received a stronger prescription. I remembered how those feelings had been dismissed by my eye doctor. I had forgotten all of that in optometry school as I learned to observe the process scientifically.

Now I could see what really occurred when the typical patient got a new pair of lenses: Until then, he had been getting by okay without any glasses (or by wearing his old glasses). Yet within a few days of getting (the new) glasses he would be wearing them all the time. Whenever he would try to take them off, everything would look very blurry—much blurrier than he had ever remembered it being before. If he tried asking his doctor about it, the response would be: *"Don't worry, you'll get used to it."* Within a few weeks he could hardly see anything without the new glasses, but he wouldn't notice this because he just never tried to see without them anymore. He had become totally addicted and didn't even know it. He thought that wearing glasses all the time was normal, because his doctor had given him that impression.

A year later he would be back in the eye doctor's office, and his visual complaint would be essentially the same as it had been the year before: "I can't see the blackboard," or "I can't see the computer screen," or "I can't see to drive at night." The doctor would go through the same set of tests and questions. The patient would again plead, "Can I see number one again, please?" And the doctor's recommendations would be the same: a stronger pair of glasses.

This familiar process would repeat itself each time he saw the eye doctor. So, after years of experience with the eye-care profession, he might simply come in and say, "Doctor, I need a stronger prescription." He knew what the doctor was going to suggest, so he didn't even bother to describe his symptoms anymore.

This would happen year after year. Usually the patient never asked any questions. Only occasionally a brave patient or parent would ask, "What's going on? Johnny's eyes have gotten worse for five years in a row. Is he going to lose his eyesight?" The doctor would say, "Don't worry, Mrs. Brown. Your son has progressive myopia." But what the eye doctor didn't realize was that the vision care she had been taught to practice had actually encouraged this progression.

The subject of preventive measures hardly ever came up. The patient was usually afraid to ask about it. After all, the doctor might get irritated, and embarrass or shame the patient. "What a silly question," the doctor might say. "Everybody knows you can't change your eyesight!" I can understand why the typical eye doctor would react that way. Almost all eye doctors wear glasses, and since they are trained to believe that preventive measures are impossible, very few of them have ever tried it themselves. So how would they know anything about it? To be a true healer, a doctor must be a living example of his own work. "Physician, heal thyself," the Bible says, and even today the art of healing is still primarily a function of our experience, not our knowledge or our credentials.

As I saw this pattern repeated over and over, I began to ask myself why eye doctors continue to use the same approach when eye problems just continue to deteriorate. Have you ever wondered why your eyes get weaker every year? Does this happen with any other part of the body? What if the function of another part of your body started to deteriorate? Say you were playing a lot of tennis and developed a case of tennis elbow. You might go see your doctor and say, "Gee, my elbow is stiff and it hurts when I move it." What if your doctor replied, "No problem. We'll just put it in a brace . . . *for the rest of your life"?* You'd quickly get a second opinion! But we don't think about doing that with our vision specialist. They tell us, "You have to wear glasses from now on," and we accept it as a life sentence. We've been so brainwashed that we don't even question it.

But those lenses are really little jail cells that lock our view of reality into a hard, unchanging focus that is based solely on judging and discriminating, on continually asking the question "Which is better, this or that?" But does vision only consist of the ability to recognize little black letters twenty feet away in a narrow, dark room? Does any test really measure anything other than our response to being tested? Can we really measure and "correct" our vision by testing it once a year? Or is our vision renewed with every breath, with every new awareness, just like the rest of our body?

Children know how little seeing clearly has to do with reading the eye chart. One day a young boy and his mother came to see me. A routine eye test had revealed that the boy had a mild case of myopia. The boy's eye doctor had prescribed a pair of glasses and the mother was trying to decide whether to get them. During our conversation I asked the boy to look out my window at the mountains on the far side of the valley, miles away. "How do they look?" I asked him. He replied, "I can see everything just fine. I just can't read those letters on the chart!"

One of the most potent aspects of our genetic makeup is the body's ability to continually regenerate, rebalance, and heal itself. I just couldn't understand why eye doctors thought this couldn't happen with vision. This question really hit me hard, since it was part of my own life. Why couldn't I heal my own eyes? Even though I didn't like to wear my glasses, I certainly couldn't see well enough to get by without them. In fact, I found it hard to hear without them. Sometimes I couldn't even think without them.

So I decided to go back to the basics to try to find the answer. What did I really know about vision?

Taking a Closer Look at Vision

We know that vision is by far our most important sensory channel. In fact, we receive a wider range of information through sight than through all our other senses combined—"approximately 90% of the information most of us learn in a lifetime enters through the eyes."[2] Our visual sense has three components: sensory, integrative, and motor. The sensory aspect receives information, the integrative aspect compares that visual input with our past experience and processes it through the mind's filters, and the motor aspect is the final outcome—our speech, movements, and actions. So, vision is our primary channel for learning as well as the navigational system that enables us to move through and influence our world.

Vision actually involves the entire mind/body system—it directly or indirectly affects all our thoughts, feelings, and movements. The fundamental link between vision and movement seems to be our posture, how we hold ourselves in the world. "Your vision system affects your posture—and your posture affects your vision system. Warps, gaps or lags at any point in the vision system will distort the neurological impulses going to the neck and back. Usually, such distortions lead to muscle tension." Holistically oriented optometrists have found that vision therapy can help such diverse symptoms as headaches, "chronic muscle aches, dizziness, teeth grinding, bed wetting, claustrophobia or travel sickness [that] have not responded to other help."[3] (Later sections of this book will discuss in more detail the link between how we see and how we think and move.)

The eyes are incredibly sophisticated and sensitive light receptors. A single eye contains about 1 billion working parts, which is far more complex, for instance, than a NASA space shuttle. But the most amazing fact about the eyes may be that they are actually *physical extensions* of the brain—the antennae of our cognitive network (see the figure on page 12).

The eyes are simply the externalized portion of the brain's capacity to evaluate, learn, and know. Dr. Arnold Gesell, an internationally recognized authority on child development (including the development of vision), has pointed out that "the highest acts of vision . . . belong to the supreme realm of abstract thought."[4]

When you think about it, it's just common sense that our thoughts, attitudes, and beliefs would be greatly influenced, perhaps even largely determined, by what we see in the world around us.

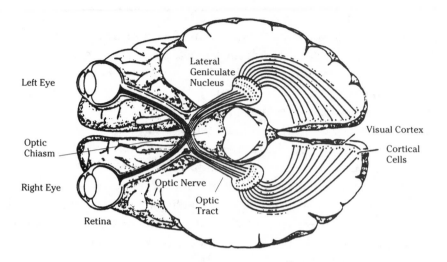

The Eyes as Extensions of the Brain (Illustration by Bunji Tagawa. Reprinted with permission of *Scientific American* from "Neurophysiology of Binocular Vision," by John D. Pettigrew, August 1972.)

However, few of us have given much thought to the opposite concept: What we see is greatly influenced, perhaps even determined, by what we believe. This perspective is not only equally valid, it is perhaps even more fundamental. The old adage "Seeing is believing" may be more accurate when reversed—"Believing is seeing."

Since mind and vision are inseparable, the most effective way to heal your vision is to start by looking into your mind. Almost every day I hear of a person who has dramatically improved his or her visual acuity by changing his or her way of thinking. The opposite is also true: Certain physical changes, such as removing corrective lenses, help us to shift our awareness. This book will show how to use both approaches.

The most powerful kind of mental shift for changing your vision is a shift of awareness. What does this mean? When we are told, "You'll have to wear glasses from now on," it's a self-fulfilling prophecy—if we believe it. We "know" that eye problems can't get better. Yet I know of many people who have experienced spontaneous, permanent visual improvement simply by realizing that it was possible, and releasing their limiting beliefs. They have learned to see in a new way by learning to think in a new way. They have learned to change their eyesight by changing their mind.

To complete that healing transformation we must turn our focus from the external world to our own feelings and experiences. Ever since childhood we've been trained to ask, "What do other people think is true?" The healing shift of awareness occurs when we replace that question with, "What is true for me?" To heal our vision we must relearn to trust the knowing that arises from within our being, rather than what we think everybody else believes.

The Quantum Mechanical Body

This transition from external authority to internal direction is also occurring in society as a whole. In the medical field, best-selling doctor/authors such as Deepak Chopra, Larry Dossey, and Bernie Siegel are radically changing some widely held assumptions about healing and illness. We are just beginning to discover the true dimensions of this new vision of ourselves, which Deepak Chopra has named the "quantum mechanical body."

Dr. Chopra, in particular, describes some fascinating new research which has confirmed that the body and the mind are not separate parts of one's being but interactive holographic fields within the whole of our awareness. Holography is a revolutionary new kind of photographic process that has the capacity to store and access enormous amounts of data. So, instead of a two-dimensional photograph, it produces a three-dimensional image—a hologram.

Most of us have seen these three-dimensional images, which can even show lifelike movement. But apart from the entertainment value of holograms, one of their most striking characteristics is that every point on a hologram contains all the information of the whole image. If you take a regular photograph and cut it into pieces, you will need all the pieces to reconstruct the whole image. However, because of its vast capacity to store data, even one tiny part of a hologram is able to re-create the whole picture. Through this book you will come to understand that *vision* is also a holographic process. I have found that vision doesn't occur at any single point in the body—such as the eyes—but throughout the body and the energy field that surrounds us.

So let's take a closer look at the new research, since its findings will form the basis for a new understanding of vision. Until quite recently, doctors believed that the mind and the body were separate functions linked by the brain, the "thinking organ," which made all of our major decisions. The brain would analyze incoming information and produce physiological reactions by sending electrical signals through the central nervous system to the body's cells.

In the 1970s this model began to be replaced due to a remarkable series of findings. The first revelation was that the brain communicates chemically, not electrically. An electrical switch has only two settings, on and off, but a chemical message can be far more complex, with subtle variations and specific shades of meaning. It soon became evident that the brain's language was far more sophisticated than we had previously suspected. According to Chopra, "The brain's vocabulary . . . [encompasses] thousands of combinations of separate signals, with no end in sight, since new [messenger chemicals] continue to be discovered at a fast rate."[5]

These newly discovered messenger chemicals were called "neuropeptides," and their job was to communicate the brain's responses—feelings, beliefs, and intentions—throughout the body. "Neuro[peptides] touch the life of every cell," Chopra says. "Wherever a thought wants to go, these chemicals must go too, and without them, *no thoughts can exist.*"[6]

It seemed obvious that these "thinking" molecules would be located in the brain, but then they were unexpectedly discovered in the immune system, which permeates every part of the body.

This was shocking. It meant that the cells of the immune system could think and feel; they could react to thoughts and feelings just like brain cells. Further research has since confirmed that when we are happy, our immune system feels happy and works with relish, and when we are sad, our immune system is depressed and far less energetic. As a result, most doctors now acknowledge that prolonged depression can weaken the immune system, and that happiness can be a powerful healing agent.

I have found that *our eyes are also made up of thinking cells,* just like every other part of the human body. When we feel sad or scared, we see in a depressed or fearful way; when we feel expansive, our vision literally "opens up."

The next discovery was even more startling: Every cell in the body creates its own neuropeptides. Every one of our cells "feels" our emotions and "thinks" our thoughts, simultaneously materializing messenger chemicals *out of nowhere* to regulate our physiological responses. The discovery that every cell contains the awareness of the whole has become the basis for a new holographic model of physiology. In the words of Deepak Chopra, "The mind has escaped the brain."[7] It also shows that the body arises out of the mind—as sages and gurus have always taught—rather than the opposite, as I learned in optometry school.

Then another chemical messenger was discovered that extended beyond the physical body. Scientists have known for years that plants, insects, and animals communicate with one another by means of "pheromones," odorless hormones that are perceived by a mysterious little gland in the nose. It turns out that humans are also constantly producing and emitting pheromones. These chemicals are triggered by our thoughts and emotions, just like neuropeptides, but are transmitted into the environment where they can be sensed by others—even after we have left the room! Invisible pheromones seem to be the subtlest form of *physical* communication yet discovered and may be a physiological explanation for our intuitive ability to sense unspoken thoughts and feelings.

Talk about nonverbal communication! We are continually releasing neuropeptides within ourselves and pheromones outside of ourselves, emanating waves of intention into the atmosphere. So, if we are sending out such clear messages, why aren't we all reading one another's minds all the time? It appears that our "gut feelings" are doing just that, but we have learned to ignore or dismiss them. I've found, however, that the more we listen for those messages, the more we are able to perceive. As Chopra often says, "Your gut feelings may be even more accurate [than your brain] because they haven't yet evolved to the state of self-doubt."[8]

The New Medicine

These ideas are very different from the beliefs that most of us were raised with and taught in school. In the words of British biologist J. B. S. Haldane, "The universe is not only queerer than we suppose, but queerer than we *can* suppose." These findings revolutionize our commonsense assumptions about the body and the mind with irrefutable evidence that the mind has not only escaped the brain but the body itself. Every cell has thoughts, feelings, beliefs, and intentions and is in constant communication with other cells, both within and beyond the skin. Furthermore, "mind" and "body" are simply different aspects of the hologram of our being, which appears to originate as "the mind" and to manifest as "the body."

In the "quantum mechanical body," any imbalances will simultaneously manifest physically, mentally, and emotionally. So what is the real cause of vision problems? Do they originate in the eyes, according to conventional medicine, or in the mind and emotions, according to this new scientific paradigm? I have found that body, mind, emotions, behavior, and environment all interact in the creation of vision difficulties. But the process really seems to *begin* when we fall out of harmonious relationship with ourselves—*when we lose sight of our relationship to the whole of life.*

This loss is often triggered by some kind of emotional stress. This stress may be the result of an obviously traumatic experience, or it may be elicited by a normal childhood event, such as a move or a new baby in the family. The biggest factor in turning this normal stress into a chronic physical symptom may be how we cope with our uncomfortable feelings. As children, did we learn to acknowledge our fear and anger and express them openly, or did we learn to suppress these feelings by somehow "changing the subject," thus disassociating ourselves from our own experience?

I have found that most of us learned very early in life to suppress our emotions rather than to feel and share them. But if we habitually ignore our feelings, they must still find expression—and it's usually in our physical body. We'll see throughout this book that vision problems often seem to be the result of a desire to *avoid looking at* some aspect of one's life.

In the old days, it was the doctor's job to fix whatever went wrong with our physical machine. We weren't expected to take responsibility for our health; we just did whatever the doctor told us to do. The new medicine requires a much higher level of commitment and participation from us.

When I graduated from optometry school, I didn't realize that what I had been taught about vision had been based on an outdated approach to healing . . . but over the last twenty years my personal and clinical experiences have led me toward a new way of seeing things—and I began to take a closer look at what I had learned.

2 What I Learned in School

Education [is] not as sudden as a massacre,
but [it is] more deadly in the long run.
—Mark Twain

HOW DOES the shift in our understanding of the mind/body relate to vision? Vision care is still overwhelmingly based on the assumptions of the old medical paradigm. Let's take a look at what I was taught in school. Most of these ideas are probably familiar to you. In fact, you may consider them to be true. However, my clinical experience (and that of hundreds of other vision specialists) overwhelmingly shows that these beliefs are actually a major source of the current epidemic of vision problems.

I was taught that vision is a mechanical function that works just like an optical lens—a "camera" in the eye. In my textbook, the chapter on the optics of the eye was preceded by a chapter on general optics. First we learned how light moved through lenses and prisms, and then we applied this to the vision process. In fact, we studied the eye as if it were a camera that just happened to be located in the head.

The ability to see clearly was called "visual acuity," which we measured as a person's ability to identify a certain size of letters at a distance of twenty feet (the standard test distance). We used twenty feet because this is the distance at which the light rays that enter the eye are roughly parallel—so it was defined as "optical infinity." In other words, looking at an object from twenty feet away is optically considered to be equivalent to looking at an object from miles or even light years away. Although this may be true for a glass lens, I've found that it is not necessarily true for the human eye, which has far greater adaptive flexibility.

In any case, "normal" vision is defined as "20/20." This number simply means that when you're standing twenty feet from the eye chart, the smallest symbols that you can read are those that eye doctors have decided a person with "normal" vision *should* be able to read at twenty feet. The first number is the testing distance (twenty feet); the second number is the distance at which a person with 20/20 vision could read that letter. As your visual acuity gets worse, the first number stays the same (because you are always tested at twenty feet) and the second number rises. For instance, a score of 20/200 means that the smallest symbols you can identify on an eye chart twenty feet away could be identified by a person with 20/20 vision at two hundred feet away.

How was this norm, upon which all lens prescriptions are based, developed? The originator of the method, Dr. Hermann Snellen, simply measured the vision of an assistant whom he felt had good eyesight, and set that as the standard against which all of us would be evaluated![1] It seems that there is no objective way to establish what ideal eyesight "should" be. So it's possible that "normal" vision is meant to be well beyond our idea of 20/20.

Corrective lenses are prescribed in diopters, which are measurements of lens power. The smallest unit is one quarter diopter. So the minimum prescription is 0.25 diopters; the higher the numbers, the stronger the lenses. A prescription of 5.50 is therefore twenty-two increments of lens power, which is a strong correction. The concave lenses that correct for nearsightedness are indicated by a "minus" prescription, such as −5.50. The convex lenses that correct for farsightedness are indicated by a "plus" prescription, such as +5.50. A lens that corrects for astigmatism (visual asymmetry) may consist of two minus corrections or a combination of plus and minus corrections.

If vision were a purely mechanical process, then it followed that the clarity of our vision could not be affected by what we saw, how we felt about what we were seeing, or how we felt about ourselves. Furthermore, since the eyes worked just like camera lenses, they certainly couldn't react or adapt to changing psychological or environmental conditions.

If our vision works like a machine and the machine isn't working, then there must be something wrong with the parts, right? Any deviation from the visual norm was called a "refractive error"—"a condition in which the eye, in a state of rest, is unable to focus the image of distant objects upon the retina."[2] (As we will see, however, in its natural state, the eye is never in a state of rest, even during sleep.) Refractive errors include conditions such as nearsightedness, farsightedness, astigmatism, presbyopia (old-age vision), and so on. I was taught that these problems were inborn flaws or limitations in the eye's equipment, and that we could only examine them by analyzing the physical structure of the eye. In this way, we had "discovered" that nearsightedness was caused by a long eyeball and farsightedness by a short eyeball.

This physical definition of vision is the basis for the two methods that most eye doctors use to determine your prescription—the "subjective" and "objective" approaches. The "subjective" method is the familiar part of the vision exam in which the doctor asks you, "Which is better, number one or number two?" It's called "subjective" because it asks you to judge the clarity of the two choices *based on your own perception.*

The "objective" method, on the other hand, is strictly a mechanical approach designed to bypass your perception completely. This method measures each eye's ability to focus light on the retina, as if it were a camera lens—how well you can actually see is irrelevant. The eye doctor begins by placing your eye at rest—either by putting a lens in front of your eye to blur your vision, or by paralyzing your ability to focus with eye drops. A beam of light is then sent into your eye and the focusing power of the eye is equalized with a series of optical lenses. (This process is called "retinoscopy.") The doctor knows the proper correction has been found when the beam of light passing through the lenses focuses directly on the retina rather than behind or in front of it.

It sounds pretty scientific, right? Unfortunately, it ignores what I have found to be some of the most important factors affecting visual acuity. It completely avoids the fact that when the eye is working properly, it is never in a state of rest but in continuous movement. As we'll be seeing later, whenever the eye stops moving, our vision begins to deteriorate. It also does not take into account that even when the eyes are in an artificially induced "resting" state, the mind/body will retain any habitual stress or tension that may have been undermining the visual acuity. Finally, this method is unable to assess true vision because, as we will be seeing later, vision is actually more of a projective process than a receptive one.

To prescribe corrective lenses, eye doctors generally use a combination of the objective ("retinoscopy") and subjective ("Which is better?") tests. However, in formal studies of vision improvement, the objective measurement is the *only* test that is considered to prove scientifically that vision change has taken place. We'll see later that the results of the two tests can be quite different, and that *both* often differ from how well we actually see when we walk outside on a sunny day.

Why? The objective approach artificially paralyzes the natural function of our eyes, ignores the link between vision and the mind, and is based on the questionable premise that objective observation is possible. The subjective test, on the other hand, only measures one tiny aspect of our vision, and it doesn't consider that the observer's beliefs and state of mind may be affecting the measurements. *Both* tests are based on the mistaken assumptions that our vision is physically determinted and that we see only with our eyes, so they block out all of the nonmechanical aspects that make our vision come alive (I'll be explaining all of this more fully later).

As a result, how well you can actually see may have very little to do with how a vision specialist would define your visual acuity. This distinction becomes especially important in defining vision improvement (or lack of improvement). For instance, although I now have vivid and clear vision (and can even see things that are considered to be invisible), an *objective* measurement of my eyes would indicate that I'm still moderately nearsighted and significantly astigmatic.

That would be enough for many eye doctors to tell me that I still require glasses, although I *don't* need them to see clearly.

So, although it is a demonstrable fact that I can see quite clearly without glasses, according to the objective measurement my vision improvement simply doesn't exist. My case is typical of that of thousands of others who can see far more clearly (or in some cases, far less clearly) than the shape of their eyeball would indicate. Conventional eye care has been able to ignore experiences such as these by defining vision improvement only as a change in the physical shape of the eye rather than as a change in how well we can see. The mechanical definition of vision says that these two must be the same, but they aren't.

As a rule, the rest of the eye-care profession has been taught the same doctrine that I was: Focusing problems (such as myopia) are due to the shape of the eyeball, and the shape of the eyeball is pre-programmed by our genes—therefore, vision improvement is impossible.

Since I went to school, eye doctors have developed surgical techniques (such as radial keratotomy) that reshape the front of the eyeball—the cornea—to improve eyesight without lenses. These radical and invasive "treatments" are the natural result of taking the mechanistic approach to its logical conclusion. Although these procedures are based on viewing the eye as just another optical system, their outcomes are surprisingly unpredictable and may even have unintended consequences. That's because what may appear on the surface to simply be a focusing problem in the eye is actually a deeply ingrained neurological pattern that affects every aspect of our behavior. Making a dramatic alteration in this pattern can be like suddenly changing a car's finely balanced steering mechanism—without telling the driver.

The conventional view of vision problems has been that, in most cases, they just aren't that significant. In the words of Dr. Ray Gottlieb, a proponent of the holistic approach, "The problem of [poor vision] is generally not considered to be a problem at all. Nearsightedness is considered a normal fact of life by most professionals and by most nearsighted people."[3]

Dr. Gottlieb goes on to point out that very little has been scientifically proven about the origin of myopia: "The research is marked by inconsistencies and much confusion. Because of the lack of conclusion and the feeling that little could be done about it, the causes of [deteriorating vision] are scarcely mentioned in professional education and students are left with the impression that, like Topsy, [these] conditions 'just growed.'" So although the research has been inconclusive, most optometrists and probably all ophthalmologists are still being taught that vision is a purely mechanical process.

If the hereditary shape of the eyeball is really the cause of weak vision, why didn't our ancestors suffer from the same problems? People do not realize that an epidemic of vision problems—especially myopia—has recently emerged in the industrialized world, while nearsightedness is still almost unheard of in less-developed societies. The incidence of myopia seems to escalate, *within one generation,* as people become more literate and spend more time indoors. Gottlieb mentions several studies that have demonstrated this effect: "Young [in 1969] found a 59 percent incidence of myopia among sixth-grade Eskimo school children, but only a 5 percent incidence in their parents and *none at all* among their grandparents." In 1964, Sato found a "two to three times increase of myopia in Japan over a twenty-five-year period which came at a time of industrialization and westernization."[4] So, although genetics may play a role, other factors are obviously involved.

Even in the modern world, "the incidence of myopia is markedly lower among peasants or farmers than among highly educated and professional people."[5] In fact, the more education you have, the more likely you are to be myopic. The statistics look something like this:[6]

Age or Educational Level	% Myopic
At birth	less than 1
age 5 to 9	3
age 10 to 12	8
end of 8th grade	20
high school graduation	40
college graduation	60–80
graduate students	80[7]

The correlation between educational level and myopia is so high that "there is even an attitude that nearsightedness is a positive adaptation in our society."[8] Why has the medical community and the general public been so unconcerned with this epidemic of deteriorating vision? Sure, we can "correct" our vision by wearing glasses or contacts, but that can also be a convenient way to simply sweep the problem under the proverbial rug. The truth is that "lenses that only work on the symptom of nearsightedness are compensating lenses; they mask the serious nature of the condition."[9] The conventional approach to vision care simply does not acknowledge the possibility of reversing vision problems; its attitude is summed up by M. J. Hirsch: "If nothing other than [correction] can be done, it is better to know this and to educate and reconcile children to the situation than to join them and their parents in a chase of will-of-the-wisps."[10]

The Chinese have found that the escalation of myopia with modern education *is* reversible, given a public commitment to vision improvement. In 1949, the Chinese government decided to do something about the increasing incidence of myopia. So Chinese students and factory workers do eye exercises twice a day, for about ten minutes, using an official poster of eye exercises. As a result, the Chinese say they have actually *reversed* their increase in myopia (see pages 26 and 27).[11]

It's hard to reconcile all these findings with the theory that unclear vision is simply due to mechanical defects in the shape of the eye. An alternative explanation was first proposed by Dr. William Bates in the 1920s. Bates was a respected ophthalmologist in New York City when he began to question the effectiveness of using corrective lenses to treat vision problems. He developed a radically new explanation of vision problems and how to treat them, which was firmly rejected by the medical establishment at the time (and ever since).

Bates's work is the foundation of the natural approach to vision improvement. He proposed that poor vision originated not in mechanical factors within the eye but in a combination of physical, emotional, and mental responses to an environment of unhealthy stress. Dr. Gottlieb points out that this holistic approach sounds amazingly up-to-date today, almost seventy-five years after it was first presented: "Modern civilization forces individuals to exist under continual strain, worried, lost in thought, reviewing memoirs of past experiences which filter out present experience. It is only within the last decade that popular attention has begun to focus on . . . stress-related illnesses, a relationship which Bates pointed out over six decades ago."[12]

As Bates himself wrote in 1920, "If [primitive man] allowed himself to get nervous, [he] was promptly eliminated; but civilized man survives and transmits his mental characteristics to posterity."[13]

Bates's opponents point out that his approach has never been "scientifically" proven to be effective—but can we really explain away the thousands of people who have benefited from natural vision improvement in the last seventy-five years as simply *imagining* that they can see without their glasses? It appears that the real barrier to widespread acceptance of Bates's method is that it is based on an entirely new way of thinking about vision. His approach is so different from the "accepted theories of physiological optics"[14]—the mechanical explanation of vision—that it may not even be testable without a new "psychophysical model" of how vision works. Gottlieb, for one, suggests that the current methods of studying changes in vision may be inadequate, which would not be surprising, in light of the accepted doctrine that vision changes are impossible in the first place.

Bates's ideas were not mentioned during my training. We did hear that "behavioral" optometrists believed that the stress of reading was the primary cause of vision problems. These doctors said that reading is a biologically unacceptable activity that creates physiological stress, affecting the structure of the eyeball. However, that theory was not given much credence by mainstream eye doctors. The main assumption was always that vision problems can't be prevented or healed. So we were simply trained to measure the problem, compare it to a standard of normal operation, and then prescribe the appropriate lenses to correct it.

The psychological aspects of vision were also hardly mentioned. Yet we've seen that vision is our most important sense, the helm of

EYE EXERCISES
from the People's Republic of China

1. Keep eyes closed while doing the exercises.
2. Fingernails should be short and hands clean.
3. Massage lighly and slowly until the area becomes a little bit sore; do not use excessive pressure.
4. Do eye exercises twice a day—once in the morning and once in the afternoon—while sitting with elbows resting on table.

EXERCISE I

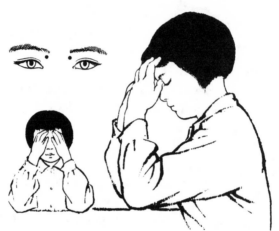

Use thumbs to massage inside eyebrow corners with other fingers slightly curled against forehead. (8 times)

EXERCISE II

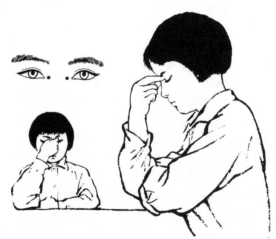

Use thumb and index finger to massage nose bridge. Press downward and then upward. (8 times)

EXERCISE III

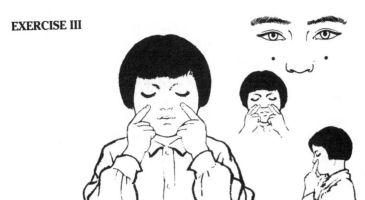

With thumbs on lower jawbone, place index fingers and middle fingers together against both sides of nose near nostrils. Then lower middle fingers and massage the cheeks where the index fingers remain. (8 times)

EXERCISE IV

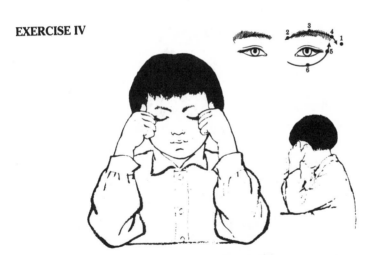

With fingers curled under and thumbs on each side of forehead, use the sides of the index fingers to rub outward following the diagram pattern: 2-3-4-6-5. (8 times)

our neurological network. What we see profoundly influences our mental/emotional state and vice versa, but you would never know that by what I learned in school!

Like most other optometrists, I was trained to administer the twenty-one-point vision examination—a comprehensive series of specialized vision tests, including the subjective and objective methods described earlier. This procedure measures almost every aspect of the visual process—in isolation—and then analyzes their relationships to one another. In real life I found that not even this battery of tests was able to evaluate *true vision,* the integrated system of how we really see in everyday life. The individual parts never seemed to add up to the whole person. However, in practice, the full twenty-one-point procedure is rarely performed anyway. So most of the time the eye doctor is only measuring a tiny portion of the patient's *eyesight,* which in turn is only one small aspect of his *vision.*

Furthermore, the standard vision exam takes place in a setting that does not even come close to the natural conditions under which our vision is designed to operate. Instead, the test environment is carefully designed to make it easier for the doctor to isolate and measure the different aspects of vision. In this test, accuracy of measurement is a higher priority than understanding the true nature of vision. This illustrates one of the unfortunate side effects of the mechanical model: the assumption that the factors we can measure numerically are the most important aspects of health. What kind of definition of vision (or life) do we get when we leave out such unmeasurable elements as insight, beauty, and well-being?

Usually, both the doctor and the patient assume that the measurements the doctor is taking have a direct relationship to how clearly the patient can see outside of the doctor's office. As we've seen, these measurements leave out the nonphysical aspects of vision—the effect of thoughts, emotions, and intentions—all of which are inseparably linked to our health, including how well we can see. Vision specialists are aware that visual acuity is not directly related to the strength of one's prescription. This is true regardless of how the prescription is measured, but the difference can be most striking when only the objective test is used (as in my case), since this method ignores our own perception of our vision. Eye doctors don't usually spend much time wondering about the difference between our natural outdoor eyesight and the measurements on which our prescription is based. They also aren't usually aware of just how large this discrepancy can be.

One optometrist, Jennifer Nelson, made this "unexplainable" difference the topic of her doctoral thesis. Citing the results of previous studies, she wondered:

> What accounts for the fact that among (those with a prescription of −1.00) uncorrected visual acuity can vary from 20/100 to 20/30 . . . ? By what means does a myopic individual with uncorrected visual acuity of 20/400 suddenly see 20/50 uncorrected during hypnosis . . . ? How is it that a (person with a prescription of −5.00) with uncorrected visual acuity of 20/800 gains the ability to see 20/30 without the aid of lenses following sensory feedback visual acuity training . . . ?[15]

More cases of our ability to see clearly regardless of our prescription strength are described throughout this book. In fact, my experience is that such changes are possible for almost anyone—*without* the aid of hypnosis or biofeedback training. My eyes, for example, still yield an objective measurement that should limit my acuity to about 20/200, and yet I usually see with a clarity *beyond* normal vision. I've known of thousands of other people who can see significantly better than their prescription would indicate. There are also many people who see far *worse* than they "should" according to their prescription.

This difference between subjectively reported visual acuity and the objectively measured prescription is actually a common phenomenon that has been observed in many studies. The problem has been that it is not usually given any validity, because it does not fit the scientific definition of clear vision—the objective measurement. For instance, one article concludes that the results of vision improvement studies (which test various techniques, including Bates's method) "have not been encouraging" because their "only advantage may be improved visual acuity."[16] Well! The author goes on to warn that even this effect may only be due to the patients' having memorized the chart, which certainly seems to be a factor the studies could have taken into account. No wonder Gottlieb suggests that we need better methods of studying vision improvement techniques.

Here and there a few researchers are beginning to recognize that some kind of nonphysical factor may be affecting vision. As one abstract explains, "The change in acuity in the absence of a refractive shift suggests sensory adaptation to blur. However, the demonstrated change in visual acuity appears to be less than that which is subjectively reported; accordingly, psychological input cannot be ruled out."[17] Or, in plain English: "Our tests showed that these people could see better than we expected them to, and the difference isn't all 'blur interpretation.' So we can't be sure that the missing link isn't some kind of psychological factor." Still, notice how cautious they are about even *suggesting* this possibility!

A New Perspective on Vision Care

Despite our vast scientific knowledge of the mechanics of the eye, the epidemic of poor vision is still spreading. Most vision specialists do not care to speculate about whether there might be anything fundamentally flawed about our approach to vision care. They simply keep prescribing corrective lenses, as they were trained to do.

Here and there, however, revolutionary new ideas are popping up around the fringes of the eye-care profession. More and more vision specialists are beginning to wonder about what they learned in school. Every once in a while they hear of a case that just can't be explained away. The most common story is of someone who used to wear glasses but stopped wearing them as much—and improved his eyesight. It's just not supposed to happen that way, but even many eye doctors have experienced something that they have been trained to believe is physically impossible. Here's the story of Larry Simons, an optometrist in California who attended one of my weekend workshops in 1986 (Larry's visual acuity had previously been tested as about 20/200):

On the first day I took off my glasses so Jacob could test my vision. As I was reading the chart he kept reminding me to breathe, and to my surprise, the symbols on the eye chart began to get clearer and clearer. We were using an unfamiliar chart that had numbers instead of letters, so I knew that I wasn't just reading it from memory. I actually read down to the 20/25 line—it was incredible!

I put my glasses back on afterwards, but later that afternoon Jacob asked me to take them off again. He examined them for a minute, and then he said, "You don't need those." I said, "Yes, I do." He said, "No, you don't." He refused to give them back to me! He finally did return them a few hours later, and as I put them back on he asked me, "How do they feel now?" I noticed that they felt really tight—I couldn't ever remember noticing that before. Jacob suggested that I keep my glasses off for the rest of the weekend, which I did. I was surprised to discover how comfortable I could get without glasses in just one weekend. At the end of the workshop I drove home—from San Diego to Los Angeles—with my glasses on the seat beside me instead of on my face.

Now, more than six years later, my acuity is right around 20/40. I don't wear glasses. I see everything that I want to see and do everything that I want to do without them. I play sports, practice optometry, and drive twenty-five miles each way to and from work. I don't worry about glasses. This is a much nicer way to live.

So, do glasses really help us to see better? Or do they keep us locked into a tiny fraction of our visual and emotional range?

I have found—from my own experience and that of thousands of other people—that if you really want to see clearly, take off your glasses! The next few chapters will describe how I improved my vision from about 20/200 to beyond 20/20, and the rest of the book is a guide to improving your own vision. After twenty years of clinical experience with vision improvement, I know that any motivated person can do what I did.

It all started with a simple experiment.

3 An Experiment on the Workings of the Mind

It isn't that they can't see the solution.
It is that they can't see the problem.
—G. K. Chesterton

THE SURPRISES I found in my first years of practice had raised a lot of questions. Can we really assess vision by doing an eye examination, or is there more to vision than meets the eye? Is vision limited to the eyes, or even the brain? Is it merely a means of navigating in the physical world? Does vision come from the outside in or emanate from the inside out? I wondered if we really knew the answers to these questions, or if anyone else was asking them. If they were, they were apparently keeping it to themselves. None of my colleagues appeared to be interested in these questions, and I knew no one else who I could discuss them with.

By early 1976, I decided that I had to do *something* to find some answers. I especially wanted to know if there was a relationship—and if so, what it was—between vision and the mind. Many books were beginning to come out about the link between the mind and the body, but I wasn't much of a reader, and I realized that I could do my own experiment by observing myself. I called my exploration "an experiment on the workings of my mind." I had the idea from accessing various meditative states that there must be a "clear vision button" somewhere in my head. If I could just locate this button with my awareness, I would be able to shift the part of me that couldn't "see what was going on," and my vision would open up.

Every afternoon, around the time parents were picking their chil-

32

dren up from school, there was a slow period in the office. I decided to use this time for my experiment. We had a vision therapy room where we worked with children who had visually-related learning problems. I decided to go in there every afternoon and take my glasses off for a while, just to see what would happen. The first day I sat down, removed my glasses and placed them on the table next to the chair. Then I just sat there and looked around. Nothing seemed to be happening. As I was sitting there, my right hand very quietly reached over, grabbed my glasses, and put them back on my face! I didn't even realize what I was doing. Before I knew it, I was back working in the office, as usual.

The same thing happened the next day and the day after that. Every day I would go into the room, remove my glasses, and, after a few minutes, unconsciously slip them back on. After several days of this, I noticed an uneasy, anxious feeling that seemed to arise just before I reached for my glasses. I tried to wait a little longer, past the point when I noticed the discomfort. The longer I waited, the more uneasy I became. The uneasiness turned into anxiety. The anxiety turned into fear. The fear turned into other emotions—sadness, anger, or feeling out of control. The longer I kept my glasses off, the more feelings would surface. As soon as I put them back on, the feelings disappeared. Trying to make sense of this, I vaguely wondered if I could be using my glasses to modify my emotional state, just as an alcoholic uses alcohol. This was my first inkling of just how addictive those little lenses are.

One day, after my glasses had been off for about fifteen minutes, I was wondering how merely removing a pair of corrective lenses could create such powerful emotions. Then it dawned on me that I had it backward: The glasses were masking my awareness of the uncomfortable feelings. These feelings, then, must be aspects of my life that I *couldn't bear to see*. I had blurred them out and then unknowingly buried them by wearing glasses. The longer I kept my glasses off, the more they would keep surfacing. This theory fit my experience, but could it be possible? None of my teachers in optometry school had mentioned any connection between vision and emotions.

As I sat with my glasses off a few days later, I looked up from my chair and glanced at the eye chart at the other end of the room. It looked different somehow. Then I realized that I was clearly seeing the 20/80 and 20/70 letters, which are about half the size of the 20/200 letters—the best I'd been able to see in years! I couldn't believe it. I was so excited! I couldn't wait to share the miraculous news with my colleagues. I said to one of them, "I've been doing this experiment, and my vision is twice as good as before!" He gave me a strange look and said, "That's just blur interpretation," as if to say, "How could you be so naive?" All the other optometrists whom I shared this experience with responded in the same way. I felt like a child who had been slapped in the face. They didn't even want to hear about the experiment. After all, I didn't have a control group or a statistically significant study—I was just recording my own experiences.

I continued anyway, slowly extending the time that I would sit there, and my vision just seemed to get better and better. The longer I kept my glasses off, the more clearly I could see. Eventually I decided to reexamine my prescription. After all, if the vision tests could measure eyesight that was deteriorating, they should also be able to measure eyesight that was improving. If this experience was real, and not just a figment of my imagination, my prescription should be measurably weaker.

I sat myself down in the examination chair and placed that large instrument in front of my face. I did the complete series of tests on myself, and it was very enlightening. For the first time I asked *myself* that famous question, "Which is better, number one or number two?" How confusing it was to be both the patient and the doctor at the same time!

It also seemed strange that this large optical instrument was totally blocking my visual field. I knew that the eyes process visual information both centrally and peripherally. *Central* vision is whatever we are focusing on; it perceives the details and colors of the stationary objects in our central focus. Our central vision is primarily active during the day, as it works best under high levels of illumination. *Peripheral* vision enables us to perceive shapes and movement. It scans the objects out to our sides around our central focus. We use peripheral vision at all times, and it is our primary form of perception in the dark, under the lower light levels of night-time. Yet here I was in a totally dark room, where I should be using my peripheral vision, but it was being totally blocked by a large optical instrument. I realized that my prescription was being based on my confused responses to a series of questions that just didn't feel right. My guts kept trying to tell me that this whole setup just didn't make sense.

Despite this sense of disorientation, when the exam was completed, I found that my prescription actually *was* weaker than before. Even though I didn't like wearing glasses, I was so thrilled about the weaker prescription that I couldn't wait to get my new lenses. In the meantime, I continued to wear my old lenses less often—whenever I noticed that I didn't really need them, I would take them off.

Then the new lenses arrived and I put them on—and something very unexpected happened. As soon as I put the frames over my face, it felt as if my whole being was shrinking inward. My eyes felt very tight, almost painfully so. My awareness seemed to be pulled inside, and the vital energy flowing through my solar plexus seemed suddenly cut off. What in the world was going on?

Seeing the World Through a Hole

Since I hadn't been wearing my glasses as much, when I suddenly put them on again, I felt a dramatic shift in my perception. The same narrowing and tightening effect actually occurs every time we put on corrective lenses, but we usually become so accustomed to it that we stop noticing it. You may remember a similar feeling the first time you put on a pair of lenses or even when you got a stronger pair of lenses. It's the same part of your awareness that says, "Gee, this feels funny." We usually suppress our perception of that discomfort because we trust our doctor's words: *"Don't worry, you'll get used to it."*

When I put those glasses on, I began to discover the real difference between seeing with glasses and seeing without them. We usually think we don't see as clearly without our corrective lenses, but what we think of as seeing less clearly is actually just seeing differently. I noticed how the glasses seemed to reproduce the effect of the long, narrow testing room in front of my face. They seemed to constrict my peripheral vision, just as I had experienced during the eye exam. They also seemed to limit me to one narrow way of seeing and thinking, based on analytical judgment. It was as if I was always asking, "Which is better, this or that?" about everything I saw. Ray Gottlieb, the holistic optometrist, describes this analytical mode as composed of two mental processes—categorizing ("What is it?") and reasoning ("What is to be done?")—that we use in order to focus our attention, especially when we feel endangered.[1] I simply noticed that I couldn't *feel* my world or perceive its wholeness while my awareness was so focused. I began to wonder: Are there areas of perception that we miss when wearing lenses that are more important than seeing details more clearly?

How did putting on a pair of lenses create this feeling of constriction? I was familiar with studies which indicated that the two aspects of vision weren't simply about seeing straight ahead and seeing out to the side.[2] Central vision, on which all the routine tests are focused, is the aspect of our mind's eye that looks analytically, that scrutinizes the details of our world. Peripheral vision, which is rarely examined unless pathology is suspected, is the aspect of our mind's eye that *feels* the world *as a whole.* This global perspective enables it to continuously scan the entire range of our perceptive field and decide what to bring into focus next.

The peripheral aspect of our vision is significantly reduced when we wear glasses. Remember how the optometrist puts that little ruler across your nose? She is measuring the distance between your pupils so that the optician can place the exact prescription directly over the center of each eye. If you examine your glasses carefully, you may be able to locate this optical center. The problem with this standard lens design is that it doesn't take into account the fact that your eyes are in constant motion. Your prescription actually changes every time your eyes look away from the optical center. Your eye doctor doesn't mention this, because her training gave her the impression that it wasn't important.

How important is it? When you look through the full prescription at the exact center of your glasses, you can discriminate very well. You can see all the details as if you're looking through a microscope or a telescope. As soon as your eyes move right, left, up, or down—*anywhere* other than straight ahead—your prescription shifts and the details begin to lose their focus. A prismatic effect is created that distorts the clarity of your vision. Your eyes respond to this distortion by repeatedly returning to center and eventually deciding to stay there.

By encouraging us to only look straight ahead, those glasses become a highly effective feedback tool that trains the eyes to remain in one position—they literally teach us to view reality through a single fixed point of view. However, the part of our vision that looks straight ahead only knows how to analyze and discriminate. The more we wear our glasses, the more we learn to judge our world rather than feel it, the more we lose our innate ability to sense its wholeness.

The Keys to the Mind

The feedback created by corrective lenses not only blocks our peripheral vision, it also limits the range of our eye movements. We don't usually think of the tiny movements of the eyes as anything important, but as we move our eyes less, we actually reduce our capacity to access our feelings. How does this happen? Psychologists have noticed that in order to access specific types of data or memories in our brain, we must move our eyes in a particular direction.

Here's an experiment to get an idea of how this works. I suggest that you do it without your lenses on, as the effects will probably be clearer that way. You can do it by yourself, but it may be easier if you work with a partner. If you're working alone, silently answer the following questions while noticing how your eyes move as you locate the answer to each. If you're working with a partner, read the questions to the other person and observe how their eyes move as they answer each question (they don't need to say the answers out loud):

- What was the color of your first bicycle?
- What would your mother look like with bright green hair?
- What does it feel like to stroke a kitten?
- What does the National Anthem sound like?

You will notice that each question elicits a specific eye movement or combination of movements—up, down, left, right, and so on. These movements are the keys that open the mind's "file cabinet" to locate the file "color of first bicycle," or whatever information you are seeking. There is no "correct" direction to move your eyes, but most people have a predictable pattern of movements, depending on the nature of the information they are trying to retrieve. In my case, I look to the upper left to get "color of first bicycle," and to the upper right to get "mother with green hair." To remember what it feels like to stroke a kitten, I look to the lower right, and to remember the tune of the National Anthem, my eyes move straight across to the left.

All our past experiences are stored in these file cabinets, and we instinctively know that we can suppress painful or uncomfortable memories by immobilizing our eyes. Wearing glasses tends to suppress our natural eye movements, and we also often develop the habit of substituting head movements for eye movements. These habits keep the difficult feelings evoked by our memories locked within the cabinet, but excessive head movement also creates unnecessary tension in the neck and shoulders and may even encourage the development of astigmatism. Since what you don't use, you lose, this habit causes the unused eye muscles to steadily become more rigid and inflexible. At the same time, we tend to lose touch with our emotional authenticity.

Many people ask me, "What about contacts? Aren't they better than glasses? No matter which way they turn, your eyes are always looking through the center of the contact lens." However, that's also the main problem with contacts: If you wear them all day (as most people do), your eyes *never deviate* from the single focus that the eye doctor prescribed. With glasses, the eyes at least have the possibility of wandering away from the optical center. Contacts are also more difficult than glasses to take on and off as you need them. Because they are harder to use only when you need them, some longtime contact lens wearers find that switching to glasses is a key step in weaning themselves from corrective lenses. Others prefer to switch to disposable soft lenses and gradually decrease their correction. I find that although they may be more difficult to use therapeutically, for some people contacts can be a useful transition to a weaker prescription.

Freezing Your Vision

All corrective lenses discourage, and eventually cripple, visual flexibility. You could say that they waste our eyes' most precious talent. The eyes can only see clearly by continuously moving and adapting to differing distances, light conditions, etc. Whenever we immobilize the eyes by staring or fixing our focus, we begin to see less clearly. Here's an easy exercise that demonstrates what happens when the eyes stop moving: Take off your glasses or contacts. Look up from the page and gaze at a point or object that you can see relatively clearly. Fix your eyes there; don't allow them to move. Continue staring at that point without blinking until your vision changes. What happens to your visual clarity and your visual field as you continue to stare? Most people find that their visual clarity begins to deteriorate and their visual field begins to shrink and dim when they stare for a prolonged period of time.

It is natural for the eyes to keep moving. In fact, they really only stop moving when we interfere with their normal function by trying to see. Whenever we focus intently on something, our vision blurs and the visual field closes in. This simple fact is enormously important in understanding and healing vision difficulties. It is the basis of the Bates Method, the first system of natural vision improvement. William Bates believed that poor vision began with unhealthy habits of seeing created by mental and emotional tension: "Mental strain of any kind always produces a conscious or unconscious eyestrain, and if the strain takes the form of an effort to see, an error of refraction is always produced. . . . Unfamiliar objects produce eyestrain and a consequent error of refraction because they first produce mental strain."[3]

Could that be why so many people feel that their vision actually deteriorates during an eye exam? Dr. Bates relates an example: "A schoolboy was able to read the bottom line of the [eye chart] at ten feet, but when the teacher told him to *mind what he was about* he could not see the big C, which is normally read at two hundred feet. . . ."[4]

The novelist Aldous Huxley had a miraculous recovery from near-blindness using the Bates Method. He went on to write *The Art of Seeing,* an excellent book on vision improvement. Huxley describes the process that leads to defective vision as follows:

> In our over-eagerness [to see] we unconsciously immobilize the eyes . . . we begin to stare at that [which] we are trying to perceive. But a stare always defeats its own object; for [clear sight] depends on the uninterrupted mobility of the sensing eyes and the mind.
>
> Moreover, the act of staring . . . is always accompanied by excessive and continuous tension . . . [so] normal functioning becomes impossible. . . . To overcome the effects of impaired functioning, the [person] stares yet harder, and consequently sees less with greater strain. And so on, in a descending spiral.[5]

Corrective lenses, especially contacts, freeze our eyes into a fixed focus that is applied to every visual task—a focus that is determined by our worst-case visual need. Do we really need the same prescription strength to drive on a dark night as we do to read a book on a sunny beach? No! When you wear contacts all day, your eyes spend every waking hour in the focus that the eye doctor determined by asking you the questions that your body didn't understand in the first place. (Some holistic optometrists will prescribe bifocals to give you a weaker correction for close-up work than for distance vision. This is a step in the right direction.)

As Huxley puts it, "The wearing of spectacles confines the eyes to a state of rigid and unvarying structural immobility. In this respect artificial lenses resemble not crutches . . . but splints, iron braces and plaster casts." If you broke your leg, would you wear a splint or a brace on your leg for the rest of your life? The longer that we wear corrective lenses, the more our eyes lose their unused range and flexibility, and the less we can see without our visual braces.

It doesn't stop there. Our mind/body immediately translates this visual constriction into emotional, mental, and energetic narrowing. We become psychologically stuck in a fixed view of the world as a collection of little details. Our mind's eye begins to embody the old-world view: "Don't feel anything. Don't express anything. Don't think for yourself. Just follow the rules." Our visual "crutches" seem to be perfectly designed to adapt us to life in the old paradigm, and as long as we wear them, it becomes much more difficult to break free of our self-limitations.

4 Open Focus:
Let Your Vision Escape Your Eyes

You see, but you do not observe.
—Sherlock Holmes

NOW THAT I realized just how uncomfortable my glasses really felt, I was even more motivated to spend as much time as I could without them. I was now spending about thirty minutes every day without glasses, so I began to lengthen the time without them and started doing some of my daily activities that way. After three or four weeks of this, I reexamined my eyesight—once more using the standard procedure of sitting behind the testing device and asking myself, "Which is better, number one or number two?" The test measurements showed that my vision had improved again! I could see even better than the month before. So again I reduced the strength of my lenses.

A month later I seemed to be seeing even more clearly, but when I retested myself, I was surprised to discover no change in my prescription. This was really confusing, because I firmly believed that the only way to show that my vision was improving was to require a weaker prescription. Even more puzzling was that it seemed my vision had actually deteriorated *during the eye exam.* What was going on? I began to wonder whether the test conditions could have created a state of physiological stress that had reduced my ability to see clearly.

Although my prescription wasn't weakening, I continued to

increase the time until I was spending the whole day without glasses. I wasn't seeing 20/20, but I could see well enough to know if my patients were reading the eye chart correctly. However, I just didn't know what to make of the experiment at this point. The test instruments were telling me not to believe my own eyes. Everything I had been taught said that I couldn't possibly be seeing better and still have the same old prescription, and yet I was. The contradiction between my beliefs and my actual experience seemed impossible to resolve. I didn't know that what I was about to discover would radically alter all my core beliefs, and not just about vision.

It all started one day when I felt very brave and decided to try to drive without my glasses. I couldn't believe it: I did just fine! I didn't even get close to another car. My prescription still hadn't changed, but I didn't even care—it felt so freeing just to be able to drive and work without glasses after all those years.

A few days later, as I was driving to work without my glasses, I began to get a terrible pounding headache. This was unusual, because I rarely get headaches. Then a few minutes later the throbbing pain suddenly disappeared. As I began to wonder why the headache had gone, it returned just as suddenly. It continued to come and go, and I realized that I must be doing something that was creating and releasing the pain. For one thing, whenever I tried to analyze it, the headache would get worse. So as I drove along, I experimented with different states of mind until I was able to stay pain-free for longer and longer periods of time. Then suddenly I realized that my vision was crystal clear. I could see every little detail, and everything I saw seemed to be vibrating with life—the air itself seemed to be filled with scintillating particles of energy. After a few minutes in that state, my headache was completely gone. I arrived at work feeling wonderful.

I didn't know what had happened. It felt as if I had been seeing from somewhere just outside my head. I described it to one of my colleagues, and he said that it sounded as if I should have my eyes checked to eliminate any possibility of a medical problem. It didn't feel as if there was anything wrong with my eyes, and I had been learning to trust my own experience more and more. Every time I got into the car I tried to re-create this state. I named it Open Focus®,* because it expanded my visual field just like a wide-angle lens. It also felt as if my point of perception was not fixed at my physical eyes.

Usually, vision is like a searchlight. Like most people, I had always focused on one thing in life. At different times it had been professional success, making money, or finding the right partner. Yet when I was looking for one thing, I was missing everything else. It always seemed that the truly important experiences—the *miracles*—were always those that I wasn't looking for. I figured that if looking at one thing caused me to miss the rest, then maybe by looking at *nothing* I would be able to see *everything*.

Open Focus is the way to look at nothing and see everything. It dissolves the normal distinction between what we think we *are* looking for and what we think we *aren't* looking for. It allows our eyes to be automatically drawn to that part of the visual field that is calling for attention at that moment. Usually it's not what we would otherwise be focusing on.

Try this: Remove your glasses or contacts. (It's much more difficult to do Open Focus while wearing corrective lenses.) Now look up and find a point of focus. For just a moment, fix your vision and focus really hard. Then relax your gaze and look at it very softly. Notice that the more intently you focus, the less you can see. You may notice that when you focus really hard, your peripheral vision dims and shrinks.

Now look at the same object without focusing or staring. Become aware of your breath and your body. Notice how your eyes feel— tired, tense, numb? Breathe deeply and release any tension in your body. Allow your visual focus to soften and expand until you see not only the first object but everything around it. Then notice how

---

*Open Focus is a proprietary trademark of Biofeedback Computers Incorporated. I have recently discovered that this term is trademarked by Dr. Les Fehmi, who has been using it for years. His approach is similar to mine, although he does not emphasize the visual aspects of Open Focus. You can contact him to order a handbook and audiotapes to assist you in entering a state of Open Focus (see Appendix A).

you can expand this even further to see everything in your visual field, still without focusing on anything in particular, and allowing your eyes to move freely.

Everything you see looks equally important. Now your eyes can direct your attention to whatever is really most important.

Although you may not notice any change in the clarity of your vision right away, Open Focus is the effortless way that your eyes were meant to see. As you practice Open Focus, notice how your eyes are continuously moving, never still. These eye movements are the instinctive dance of vision, searching out anything that needs your attention in the dynamic flow of life. Open Focus is always leading you to the next aspect of life that needs to be looked at—you never have to ask yourself, "What should I do next?"

Why do we normally look with fixed, intense concentration (which is increased by habitually wearing corrective lenses)? Why do we work so hard at something that is so easy? For one thing, as children, we are taught to concentrate, to try harder. When we do that, our eyes tighten, our vision contracts, and we see less—so we have to look even harder. It's the "descending spiral" that Huxley described—"malfunctioning and strain" that begins either with "trying too hard to do well, or by feeling unduly anxious about possible mistakes."[1] To try harder we must focus harder. As we focus harder, we begin to overuse our central vision, the aspect of our mind's eye that judges and analyzes. Practicing Open Focus allows this relentless analyzing to give way to a *feeling* sense that actually allows us to see and understand far more than before.

The effect of Open Focus is the opposite of the contraction that occurs whenever you put on glasses or contacts. I have found it to be almost impossible for you to open your focus while wearing corrective lenses, because the testing procedure on which prescription lenses are based requires you to *narrow* your focus. Open Focus reverses the habitual shrinking and tightening effect of wearing lenses. It expands and relaxes all levels of awareness—visual, mental, physical, emotional, and energetic.

Artists have always known about Open Focus. Everyone knows how an artist will periodically step back and gaze at her work. Have you ever wondered what she is looking at? Actually, she isn't looking *at* or *for* anything in particular. She is simply opening her focus, softening her awareness, allowing her vision to scan the work as a whole. She knows that in an open gaze her eyes will automatically be drawn to the spot that is out of the flow, that needs more attention. When she steps back and her eyes don't get stuck anywhere, the work is finished.

Open Focus can also be called "nonjudgmental seeing," because it is a way of seeing that gives equal importance to everything that you can perceive. You not only see the people and objects on which you normally focus, but also the "unimportant" things that you might pass right over when you're looking analytically—including yourself, the viewer! How often are you aware of yourself in your normal way of seeing? In Open Focus, as in meditation, you see without separating the observer from that which is being observed. You can even merge your awareness with what you see. For instance, if I'm looking in your direction, I may not know whether I'm me looking out at you, or whether I'm you looking in at me. My vision may appear to be emanating from within your eyes.

You might like to try Open Focus with a friend to experience this for yourself. Pick a time and a place where you won't be interrupted. Sit down facing each other; get comfortable. Don't "try" to look at each other or to create any specific effects. Just notice what happens when you are fully present in Open Focus with someone else. Give yourselves several minutes to practice in silence, and then share your experiences.

In Open Focus, neither the person you are looking at nor the wall behind him have more intrinsic importance. Whatever your eyes are being gently drawn to is most important at that moment, and your attention is constantly moving. As playwright John Osborne says, we tend to "spend [our] time mostly looking forward to the past." Regular practice of Open Focus is a great way to develop present-moment awareness, which keeps us fresh, open, and flexible. In Open Focus, as soon as you stray from the present you will find your eyes stuck on one spot, and you can use that as a signal to shift back into open attention. As with other forms of meditation, even a few minutes of practicing Open Focus each day can provide a fresh perspective on your familiar experiences.

Becoming the Sky

When I first discovered Open Focus, I was meditating every day. Sometimes I would lose myself in deep meditation—my awareness would seem to just disappear. During one of these deep meditative states, I had a very profound and startling experience. Although my eyes were closed, I could suddenly see everything—the whole room and myself in it—and I couldn't tell where I was seeing from! I wasn't seeing from my eyes or from any single point of view. I seemed to be seeing everything from everywhere. There seemed to be eyes in every cell of my body and in every particle surrounding me. I could simultaneously see from straight on, from above, from below, from behind, and so on. It felt as if I had *become the sky.*

Where do we see from and who does the seeing? *Is there* really a single part of ourselves from which vision originates? In this meditative experience, as in Open Focus, there seemed to be no observer separate from what was seen. There was simply awareness. Every cell within and without me contained the sight of the whole. As my being merged into this multidimensional visual network, I had a quantum leap of insight: We don't see with our eyes!

In a flash, this experience transformed all my concepts about vision; but it was just the beginning.

After the meditation, I returned to my normal way of seeing—through my eyes—but I could still see with amazing clarity. I was afraid that this miracle sight would leave as quickly as it had come, so I drove to my office eager to check my vision right away. I went into the examination room, but before sitting down behind the test instrument, I put up the eye chart and read every letter perfectly down to 20/15—beyond "normal" vision!—for the standard twenty-foot distance. Of course, I knew the standard chart pretty well, but I also had a large supply of research charts with all kinds of unfamiliar letters. I kept projecting them, one by one, until I was absolutely certain of the results. Yes, there was no doubt about it: I *was* seeing with perfect clarity. I had experienced a complete remission of my myopia and astigmatism.

Then I sat down behind the testing instrument. What happened next was a big shock. I did all the standard tests on myself, as usual, and . . . came up with the same prescription I had before! According to the eye exam, I still had significant amounts of near-sightedness and astigmatism, and yet I had read every eye chart in the office perfectly! I was flabbergasted. How could that be possible? If my prescription was the same as before, how was I seeing the chart? In the immortal words of Sherlock Holmes, once you "have eliminated the impossible, whatever remains, *however improbable,* must be the truth." The only explanation was that my vision had escaped my eyes.

I had no idea how my vision had expanded in that way, and it was several years before I realized that vision doesn't really occur in any single location. The ability to see is present throughout the greater whole of the mind/body. Jacques Lusseyran, a French writer, philosopher, and Resistance fighter whose eyes were completely destroyed in a childhood accident, also experienced this phenomenon. Shortly after his accident he discovered that he could still see, *even though his eyes had been completely destroyed.* In his autobiography, *And There Was Light,* he tells what happened after the bandages were removed:

> The people around me . . . told me that to be blind meant not to see. Yet how was I to believe them when I saw? Not at once . . . for at that time I still wanted to use my eyes. I followed their usual path. . . .
>
> Finally, one day . . . I realized that I was looking in the wrong way. . . . I was making something . . . like the mistake people make who change their glasses without adjusting themselves. I was looking too far off, and too much on the surface of things. . . . I began to look more closely, not at things but at a world closer to myself. . . .
>
> I saw light and went on seeing it though I was blind . . . this was not magic for me . . . but reality. I could no more have denied it than people with eyes can deny that they see. . . .[2]

As I walked along a country road bordered by trees, I could point to each one of the trees on the road, even if they were not spaced at regular intervals. I knew whether the trees were straight and tall, carrying their branches as a body carries its head, or gathered into thickets and partly covering the ground around them. . . .

According to many traditions of the occult, man has a third eye, an inner eye . . . located in the middle of his forehead. . . . [The scientist] Jules Romains [has] demonstrated the existence of visual perception outside the retina, situated in certain nervous centers of the skin, particularly in the hands, the forehead, the nape of the neck and the chest. I hear that more recently this kind of research has been carried on with success by physiologists, especially in the U.S.S.R.

But whatever the nature of the phenomenon . . . its effects seem to me much more important than its cause.[3]

Lusseyran's experience is confirmed by the story of "Sarah," as recounted by Larry Dossey in his book *Recovering the Soul*.[4] Sarah awoke from anesthesia after a gallbladder operation, during which her heart had stopped, with "a clear, detailed memory of the frantic conversation of the surgeons and nurses during her cardiac arrest; the OR layout; the scribbles on the surgery schedule board . . . ; the color of the sheets covering the operating table; the hairstyle of the head scrub nurse; the names of the surgeons in the doctors' lounge . . . who were waiting for her case to be concluded; and even the trivial fact that her anesthesiologist . . . was wearing unmatched socks."

Although Sarah's nurse commented that "strange stories" were not uncommon after anesthesia, the most amazing aspect of Sarah's case was that she had been completely blind since birth! Her experience had vividly demonstrated to her that "there's more than one way to see. . . . My vision cannot be completely in my body . . . and it cannot really all be in my eyes and my brain. When my body was least functional during the [cardiac] arrest my senses were most functional!"

Lusseyran and Sarah were able to *see* even though their eyes were blind. There are also people with perfectly functioning eyes who nevertheless *can't see*. In his fascinating book *Catching the Light: The Entwined History of Light and Mind*, the physicist Arthur Zajonc describes the surprising difficulties encountered by individuals who did not learn to see as children and first recovered their sight in adulthood:

In his systematic study of sixty-six case histories of the recovery of sight in those born blind, M. von Senden concluded that innumerable and extraordinary difficulties need to be overcome in learning to see. The world does not appear to the patient as filled with the gifts of intelligible light, color, and shape upon awakening from surgery. The project of learning to see *inevitably leads to a psychological crisis in the life of the patient,* one that can end with the *rejection of sight.*

Zajonc concludes that "the optically healthy organ of the eye alone is insufficient for sight. . . . Without an inner light, without a formative visual imagination, we are blind. . . . To give back sight to a congenitally blind person is more the work of an educator than of a surgeon. . . . The light of the mind must flow into and marry with the light of nature to bring forth a world."[5]

This "light of the mind" is an ancient belief that the eyes actually *emanate inner light* as well as absorb outer light. In the ancient world, Zajonc says, "to see was to illumine." In the words of the great German writer, philosopher, and scientist Johann Wolfgang von Goethe, "The eye is formed by the light and for the light *so that the inner light may emerge to meet the outer light.*"[6] I believe that some kind of two-way exchange of energy is closer to the true basis of vision than the mechanistic explanations of conventional vision science.

Like Lusseyran and Sarah, as long as I thought that I could only see with my eyes, I was limited to the physical aspect of my vision. However, we've seen how little of our ability to see really is physical. When my awareness expanded, I spontaneously accessed my whole vision. My eyesight became perfectly clear, although my eyeballs retained their "myopic" shape. So instead of looking only at one tiny window of our vision (our eyes), let's step back and view the whole picture—the *web of life.*

Seeing the Whole: The Web of Life

We've seen that one of the most intriguing aspects of a hologram is that each point within it contains all the information of the whole—

a hologram is actually an infinite series of wholes within wholes. From a holographic perspective, our entire field of awareness is one system (including the mind/body) that is in turn an element within an even greater whole, which I call the *web of life*. This web of life is a vast energy network that seems to surround and permeate everything. It can also be thought of as the vital energy of the life force.

Although mainstream science has traditionally dismissed the existence of energy fields, a growing number of scientists are now questioning this deeply held belief. Probably the strongest hypothesis for a new scientific model involving energy fields has been made by the biologist Rupert Sheldrake. In 1981 he proposed a radical and far-reaching new theory to account for several "unsolved biological problems." Among other questions, Sheldrake was trying to explain the nature of life itself. Very simply, he proposed that "the form, development and behavior of living organisms are shaped and maintained by 'morphogenetic fields.' These fields are molded by the form and behavior of past organisms of the same species through *direct connections across both space and time.*"[7] In other words, all members of a given species are linked by an invisible network that enables them to evolve and learn as one entity.

This hypothesis flies in the face of currently accepted fundamental beliefs, not only of biology but of the entire basis of scientific materialism. As a result, Sheldrake's theory generated tremendous controversy in scientific circles, with the established opinion clearly opposed to him. Yet his ideas could not simply be dismissed. In the words of one reviewer, "Wild as they seem, Sheldrake's ideas are difficult to refute on logical grounds."[8]

His hypothesis, however, was quite testable, and several studies have been done to determine its validity. Many of them have produced statistical results that clearly substantiate Sheldrake's theory, and are difficult to explain in any other way. As early as 1983, the British journal *New Scientist* wrote that Sheldrake's theory "challenges much of modern science and has raised ire in many scientists. But evidence grows that the 'hypothesis of formative causation' may be correct."[9] Still, despite convincing research results, it has not yet been accepted by the scientific establishment.

From my own perspective, the theory of morphogenetic fields makes a lot of sense, and I believe that it will one day be accepted as scientific fact. Each generation does seem to be born with a (dormant) understanding of everything that their predecessors have learned—including all of the previous generation's beliefs and behavior patterns (which act as the curriculum for further evolution). Sheldrake's morphogenetic field seems to be one aspect of the web of life that links all of nature—and each of us seems to have our own vortex or field of energy within this network.

In my work, I have consistently observed an energy field that appears to surround every human being. What is this personal energy field? It appears to be the part (the *whole* part, holographically speaking) of the web of life within which our mind/body is embedded. It is the full awareness of our being manifested as energy. Although you may assume that you have never seen this "invisible" energy field, we'll see later in the book that most people can learn to see it. I usually observe it as a kind of aura or halo of energy surrounding the body. A process called "Kirlian photography" even allows us to photograph it. A Kirlian photograph of a finger, for instance, will show a glowing emanation around the fingertip that looks something like the sun's corona during an eclipse.

I've found that this personal energy field is our link to the greater whole, the web of life. It is the channel through which we both receive and express all of our life's experience. Just as a large radar screen can "see" farther than a small one, we both perceive and express more when the field is expanded than when it is constricted. The primary receptive frequencies through which information enters this field are our senses. So our visual field—that is, the range of our vision—is simply one manifestation of our energy field—the range of our awareness.

Why would our field contract if doing so means that we would see and hear and feel less of life? It typically happens when we feel fear or danger. Our attention contracts, and we become fully focused on the immediate threat. At that moment, we temporarily lose sight of the whole, and as a result, our being literally shrinks. I often illustrate this in my workshops by having two participants portray the postures of a blaming parent and his or her child. The person taking the stance of the parents points an accusing finger at his partner. What does the other person do? His first instinct is to run away, but if he can't do that, he will begin to collapse inward, eventually falling into a fetal position.

Dr. Gottlieb offers another illustration of how we instinctively contract our sensory awareness in response to fear:

> If a rabbit notices a potential predator, it will become alert, set up an internal plan of action (flight) and implement the plan. . . . It will run quickly to cover and will ignore any appetizing berries it comes across along its path. It thus selects which aspects of the environment to attend—the internal plan or external stimulation. Once it reaches safety and the danger has passed, it will again search the environment for potential food, sex, [etc.]. Thus it can selectively open itself up to the external environment or close itself down.[10]

When humans become afraid, our instinctive response is also to focus our attention. As our senses narrow, our energy field collapses and our physical body contracts. When apprehension becomes a chronic state with no means of escape, this habitual collapse increasingly diminishes the clarity and power of our senses. This usually reduces our conscious awareness of the fear, although its underlying intensity may actually get worse—and our body will still be aware of this even if our mind is not. We can never actually break our connection to the web of life (not even in death, apparently, according to reports of near-death experiences). However, we can, and regularly do, reduce our access to it by numbing ourselves to its continuous flow of information.

Like a radar screen, the sensitivity of our perceptive field is relative to its size. When fully expanded, it is capable of receiving a tremendous amount of information. As it contracts, it receives much less. Unlike a radar screen, however, our field is constantly fluctuating in response to our emotional state. When we are afraid, it contracts. When we feel relaxed, it expands. These fluctuations directly affect the clarity and range of our senses.

Our conscious choices to open or close our awareness are also immediately reflected on an energetic and perceptual level. Every time we suppress a perception, impulse, or feeling, our senses are temporarily diminished. When we put our glasses on—narrowly focusing our attention—we suddenly notice that we feel somehow smaller and more contracted. It's easier to notice this effect after you've had your glasses off for a while.

Although the field may contract sharply in response to a shock or trauma, it is normally self-regenerating. Yet we've seen that when we are under chronic stress, we can develop chronic energetic contraction. This process is often triggered in childhood but can occur at any age when we do not understand what is happening around us or feel unable to express our fears.

Normally, a child's field will recover as soon as she feels safe again, but many children live in a chronic state of fear or anxiety. Even in an intact and relatively happy family, the emotional pressures on children can easily begin to feel overwhelming. (Think back for a moment to your own childhood.) As adults, we tend to forget just how sensitive children are to the feelings, needs, and expectations of others. Many "normal" children live in a continual state of inner anxiety, although this may not be apparent to those around them.

While they do not describe the energy field itself, both Bates and Gottlieb believe that anxiety due to environmental stress is a major cause of myopia. Gottlieb writes:

> Prolonged and chronic involvement in such tasks as reading, or situations which are demanding but difficult to understand (e.g., family or peer group situations in which there is a demand to act "correctly" in conformity to a reality structure which the individual does not understand) can lead to chronic . . . muscle patterns and metabolic changes. *It is the thesis of this paper that myopia is one possible outcome of this behavior.* The situation of a rabbit frozen between two charging, barking dogs if repeated for a period of weeks or months would likely lead to . . . muscle contraction and metabolic changes in the rabbit which become structured into the brain and body.[11]

Under chronic pressure, the energy field repeatedly contracts and eventually collapses. Then the child's chronic fear has become a *fear of life:* a habitual state of physical, mental, emotional, and energetic contraction. In this state the child can no longer feel her painful emotions as vividly, but she can also no longer perceive her surroundings or express her feelings as fully. All of her senses have contracted to some degree, although only one or two may actually show any overt symptoms. Eventually, this state of fogginess begins to feel "normal"—and it begins to feel unsafe somehow to see, hear, or feel more fully and acutely.

Just as the energy field indicates the range and quality of our awareness, so the visual field indicates the range and quality of our visual sense. The visual field is the manifestation of our energy field that indicates not only the physical extent of our vision but also its clarity and vitality. The visual field is usually thought of as a "vision envelope" that surrounds us. Like the energy field, the visual field extends around us in all directions, but even "seeing" it in two dimensions will give you an idea of its size:

Take a moment now and stretch your arms out to both sides with your thumbs up. Look straight ahead and slowly bring your thumbs together to the front. Notice the positions at which you can first see each thumb. Those are the left and right boundaries of your visual field.

Now do the same thing with your arms extending straight up and down. Those are the vertical boundaries of your visual field.

Eye doctors are generally taught that only disease can shrink or distort the shape of the visual field, but the visual field is actually a perfect mirror of our energy field. Both fields fluctuate rhythmically—they *breathe*—in response to our feelings and experiences. In fact, due to the close connection between vision and the brain, *every* perception and experience is felt in our visual field and may affect how we see.

The size, shape, and clarity of the visual field is constantly shifting. To observe this fluctuation, keep checking your field— when you feel relaxed, when you feel stressed, when you feel energized, when you feel tired, with and without your glasses, and so on. You are likely to notice that nothing about your vision is static or fixed.

Over the years I've worked with many children who have a condition in which one eye turns inward—a crossed eye. Since they use only one eye at a time, these children have effectively shut down a large part of their visual field—they have had a serious withdrawal of their perceptive function. Many children with a turned-in eye are so energetically contracted that they are physically small for their age. In several cases, I've watched their bodies begin to expand and fill out as their visual field begins to unfold, and they literally begin to open themselves up to the world. Some of them have grown as much as six inches in six months.

Peripheral vision is the way we normally access the full range of our visual field. Since glasses tend to reduce our peripheral perception, they encourage the field to remain limited. They actually create the most common form of tunnel vision. Eye doctors are trained to look for tunnel vision only when a significant eye problem is suspected, but it actually occurs frequently in those with "normal" eyesight. I've found that many "learning disabled" children simply have a severely contracted field, resulting in tunnel vision. They're not disabled; they're simply chronically afraid. When we're that anxious, it's very hard to process information, because our perceptive network has been paralyzed. Tunnel vision is the most obvious symptom of this self-contraction. It is the result of closing off our peripheral vision—the exploratory, anticipatory aspect of our sight.

Try this: Look up from the page for a minute. As you look straight ahead, notice that you are simultaneously aware of objects to your left and right and all around you. Notice how your central vision focuses your attention on one thing. Notice how any motion on the edges of your visual field can instantly attract the focus of your attention. Peripheral vision naturally guides us to the next aspect of life that requires our attention, so it is our doorway to accessing the future.

Without our peripheral vision, we lose our sense of perspective, our ability to fit the pieces into a whole, our capacity to make sense of new information in terms of our past experience. Our self-expression is also limited, which tends to further reduce the input of new information. You can see why a child with tunnel vision must exert tremendous effort to learn even simple tasks.

Peripheral vision holds the information we need to shift our focus to whatever we will look at next. When we restrict its input (as we do when wearing glasses), we can still see straight ahead, but the rest of our perception is limited. Our options are reduced. We "can't see" the link between where we are now and where we are going next. Most of us have experienced a time when we have thought, "I wish I knew what to do next. I just don't know where I'm going. I seem to be stuck in limbo." This usually occurs when we're feeling a lot of stress. As we become stressed, we draw in our energy and lose our awareness of the periphery. We lose our frame of reference, our broad perspective on life. We stare at the elephant's tail and think we're seeing the whole animal.

At those times we may search all over for external clues, even as we instinctively sense that the answers we are seeking must be somewhere right before our eyes—if we could only find them! Eventually we find the answers—by letting go of the effort and tuning in to our own inner voices rather than by looking outside ourselves. This effortless process is very similar to Open Focus. As we gently and flexibly attend to the moment, we simultaneously remain in touch with our peripheral awareness. That subconscious "radar" is free to scan our options and is spontaneously drawn to the most resonant one. Only then do we really know where our attention needs to go next.

A wonderful illustration of the interrelationship of our attention, our emotional state, and our perceptive receptivity is provided by Jacques Lusseyran, the philosopher whose eyes were completely destroyed as a child. After he totally lost his outer (physical) vision, he found himself constantly surrounded by a luminous radiance that fluctuated with his emotional state:

> . . . at every waking hour and even in my dreams I lived in a stream of light. . . . [At times] I thought of testing it out and even of resisting it. . . . I gathered up all my energy and will

power and tried to stop the flow of light, as I might have tried to stop breathing.

What happened was a disturbance, something like a whirlpool. But the whirlpool was still flooded with light. . . . I couldn't keep this up very long, perhaps only for two or three seconds. When this was going on I felt a sort of anguish, as though I were doing something forbidden, something against life. . . .

Still there were times when the light faded, almost to the point of disappearing. It happened every time I was afraid. If, instead of letting myself be carried along by confidence . . . I hesitated . . . then without exception I hit or wounded myself. The only easy way to move around . . . was by not thinking about it at all, or thinking as little as possible. Then I moved between obstacles the way they say bats do. What the loss of my eyes had not accomplished was brought about by fear. It made me blind.

Anger and impatience had the same effect, throwing everything into confusion. . . . When I was playing with my small companions, if I suddenly grew anxious to win, to be first at all costs, then all at once I could see nothing. . . .

I could no longer afford to be jealous or unfriendly, because, as soon as I was, a bandage came down over my eyes, and I was bound hand and foot and cast aside. All at once a black hole opened, and I was helpless inside it. But when I was happy and serene, approached people with confidence and thought well of them, I was rewarded with light. . . . I always knew where the road was open and where it was closed. I had only to look at the bright signal which taught me how to live.[12]

In the same way, by allowing ourselves to follow the spontaneous turning of our awareness, we are automatically led to the next step of our life. As long as we remain relaxed, receptive, and flexibly attentive, this process occurs without any conscious effort. As soon as we become afraid or tense, it tends to shut down.

For centuries science has tried to understand vision by isolating and examining every part of the physical eye, but the mind/body is not a collection of separate parts; it is a profoundly intelligent holographic system. This intelligent wholeness is the *true source of our vision,* and seems to be the only aspect of the mind/body that science *hasn't* scrutinized.

Fragmented approaches to healing simply nibble away at the edges, leaving the core of the problem intact to manifest in another form. I've found that true healing can only arise from the whole. It seems that the underlying cause of most vision problems is a chronically collapsed field of awareness—a *fear of life*.

5 Seeing Through the Fear

We must travel in the direction of our fear.
—John Berryman

WE'VE SEEN that blind people whose physical eyes are healed through surgery invariably experience a "psychological crisis" as they *try to learn to see,* and may even fail to overcome that challenge. Emotional barriers to vision are not unique to the blind, however. Our inner world of emotions, intention, and awareness plays a profound role in our ability (or inability) to see clearly. In my workshops and seminars, I always ask the participants to reflect back on what was happening in their life in the year or two prior to the onset of their vision problem. Almost everyone I have encountered could identify an experience which triggered feelings that were profoundly difficult to deal with (at that time). Most people quickly identify a specific event (or series of events) that they feel was the beginning of their vision deterioration. They'll say things like, "I didn't want to see it," or "It was so painful that I had to blur it out."

Here are some typical examples of the kind of experiences they describe:

> At that time—shortly before I got glasses—both my parents were very ill and I had to stay with my grandparents.

> We moved, and I had to change schools. It was very different from my last school, and I just didn't feel like I fit in.

I had been living with my father, my stepmother, my sisters and brothers and then I had to move to New York to live with my mom. That was a really traumatic change, a major loss. I knew I wasn't myopic before then, because my father was an optometrist and I had regular eye exams. When I came back to visit for my next vacation, I found out that I had become myopic and he gave me my first pair of glasses.

The beginning of my myopia coincided with the time when my father abruptly and without explanation stopped coming to take me for weekend visitations.

My mom was divorced when I was about three or four. The difficult part was when she remarried; I didn't like her new husband. It was a strange time, and that is when I got glasses.

I was first prescribed glasses at age twenty as I was studying to retake my Registered Nurse examinations. I had failed my first attempt and was very upset and disappointed. I saw myself as a failure academically.

When I was thirteen years old, I was punished and humiliated in front of the whole class, although I felt I had done nothing wrong. I was so hurt that I ran all the way home. When I got home my mother said that my lips were white and I couldn't breathe. For a week I was breathless when I spoke. I was given medication and the doctor said I had a weak heart. I lost a lot of weight and was told not to take part in physical education. That's when my vision problem began.

It seems that almost any kind of perceived trauma can be the stimulus for the initial deterioration of vision. Why does a particular event trigger a chronic vision problem while another will have no obvious long-term effect? The answer is that it isn't the experience itself that leads to poor vision but our reaction to it—the coping pattern that we develop to deal with the uncomfortable feelings. When people describe a painful memory by saying, "I just couldn't bear to see what was going on," those are more than just words. On some level, these people literally averted their eyes from seeing.

We can't close off any part of our visual input without diminishing our vision as a whole. As we'll see, once this starts, it tends to become a progressive spiral of visual deterioration and emotional avoidance. For most people who wear glasses, the feelings stimulated by this initial trauma or stress are still unresolved. At first glance they may appear to be distant from our adult concerns, but on a deeper level our eyes know that we *still* can't bear to look at that memory.

Furthermore, although we all seem to carry unresolved fears within ourselves, not everyone ends up with a vision problem. Some of us tend to hold unresolved stress in our eyes, affecting our vision; others may see very clearly but be more prone to have stomach ulcers, a weak immune response, or an addiction to drugs or alcohol. A collapsed energy field will affect all aspects of the mind/body to some extent, but we generally have a few favorite locations or ways in which we manifest its symptoms—and for many of us our vision is one of those areas.

An early trauma begins a habit of "blurring out" painful experiences, which then becomes our automatic response to painful feelings. Bear in mind that the field is still capable of returning to its full expanse at any time—and will do so spontaneously whenever the fear that is distorting the field is fully released. Why do these early traumatic experiences typically trigger a spiral of emotional suppression that leads to a chronic fear of life and worsening vision problems? *The primary factors that encourage and intensify visual deterioration are the prescription lenses that are used to "correct" vision problems, the social norms that encourage us to analyze instead of feel, and the stress involved in our educational system.*

We'll be looking at all these factors in more detail later, but let's start by describing a typical process of vision deterioration:

You have an experience in childhood or adolescence that frightens or upsets you, but you don't know how to express the feelings that it has triggered. The feelings begin to get stuck inside you, and your field begins to become chronically distorted. Shortly afterward, you (or your parents or teachers) notice that you're not seeing clearly. So your parents take you to the eye doctor.

When the doctor asks you what's wrong, you say something like,

"I can't see the blackboard." You really mean, "Something has happened that is very painful. I don't know how to talk about it, and it's too scary to look at. So I'm blurring it out." The doctor is only trained to understand that you can't see, so he gives you glasses or contacts to correct your eyesight.

If you've become nearsighted, you can see more clearly up close, because your field has collapsed inward. Many nearsighted people seem to carry with them the underlying feeling "It [the outside world] is against me. I need to shrink inward to create a buffer, a safety zone, between me and the rest of the world."

If you've become farsighted, on the other hand, your self-defense has been to push your field outward, away from you, instead of shrinking it inward. Therefore you usually see things in the distance clearer. The farsighted person often seems to feel, "It's me against it [the outside world]. If I can see you a mile away, I'll be able to prepare my response before you get any closer. So I'll project my vision out as far as I can."

These responses are both forms of protection resulting from an initial shrinking of the energetic field—in one case we collapse our visual space inward, in the other we push our visual space outward. Nearsighted people follow the collapse of the energetic field with a collapse of their visual range—their primary response is caving inward, or fear. Farsighted people compensate for the collapse of their energetic field by throwing their visual range outward—their primary response is projective resistance, or anger. These two choices seem to reflect the classic stress response of fight or flight.

According to the traditional model of vision, most people will become less myopic or somewhat farsighted after age forty—they'll begin to tell their eye doctor that their "arms just aren't long enough to read anymore." This condition is called "presbyopia," or "old-age vision," and conventional theories say that it is the inevitable result of the aging of the eye. However, our vision seems to change in response to many factors, and I suspect that poor diet and environmental toxins may play a large role in the development of presbyopia. I've evaluated the vision of three men well over forty (two were in their sixties and one was in his eighties) who had perfect 20/20 eyesight at both near and far distances. The common factor among them all was that they had followed an organic vegetarian diet and "natural lifestyle" for ten to twenty years.

I suspect that an accumulation of environmental and psychological toxins gradually leads to a condition of reduced flexibility throughout the mind/body system. As a result, the eye begins to take longer to adjust its focus between near and far. The person with presbyopia usually consults an eye doctor, who prescribes eyeglasses—which seem to encourage the condition to become a permanent fixation. And yet presbyopia *can* be improved (as outlined in the next section of the book) just like any other vision problem.

Although nearsightedness may be more common in the early years and farsightedness in the later years, striking psychological and physical differences have been found between predominantly nearsighted and predominantly farsighted individuals. According to Ray Gottlieb, these differences can be best summarized as two different approaches to holding unresolved emotions in the mind/body system: "The armoring posture of the [nearsighted person] is an attitude of blocking the feeling and expression of fear, and that of the [farsighted person] is blocked rage."[1] This armoring is a kind of frozen perception that tends to trap the myopic person in the memory of past experiences, and the hyperopic person in the anticipation of future experiences.

The personality profiles that result from these two approaches are quite distinctive. The typical characteristics of nearsighted people are consistently described as "emotional inflexibility, high need for approval, avoiding confrontations, cautiousness, high tolerance for anxiety, overcontrol of emotions, low desire for change, and strong need to be 'good' and to succeed in high-status activities."[2] Physically, they are "prone to being underactive, having soft bodies, weak legs, a tense depressed chest, and a husky, breathy voice."[3] Compared to nonmyopic people, they tend to be more drawn toward "high status, academically oriented occupations, and those which appeal to an introverted, accepting person."[4]

On the other hand, farsighted people as a group are described as "extroverted and rather aggressive; they sometimes exhibit behavior problems at home and at school, are aware of their environment rather than off in daydreams, and are more easily influenced by others. Physically, they are often active, sometimes to the point of hyperactivity, have hard stiff bodies with chests overexpanded rather than underexpanded. . . ."[5]

Although these differences generally hold true, in practice the psychological distinction between nearsighted and farsighted people can be more complex than these studies indicate. I've known nearsighted people who were outgoing and neither quiet nor studious. I've also known farsighted people who were introspective and detail-oriented. However, you can generally get a quite accurate description of an individual's psychological makeup by combining information about their near- or farsightedness with other aspects of how they process visual information, which are too complex to explain here.

So let's say that you've become nearsighted and according to the eye doctor's measurements you can only see clearly eight feet away. To "correct" your vision, she will prescribe glasses that appear to extend your eyesight from eight feet out to twenty feet. You assume that the glasses have expanded your vision out into the world. But is that really true?

If you're nearsighted, take off your glasses for a moment. If you're not nearsighted, borrow a pair from a myopic friend. Hold them about a foot in front of your face. Now position the lenses so that you can see part of an object (such as the upper half of a bottle) through the lens and another part (such as the lower half of the bottle) outside the lens. This is called "splitting the target."

Notice the difference between the part of the object that you see through the lens and the part that you see outside the lens. Notice that though the image within the lens appears clearer if you're nearsighted, it also appears smaller and closer than the image outside the lens. Move the glasses closer and farther away from your eyes to see how this effect varies with distance.

Glasses haven't expanded your reality, they have collapsed it. Corrective lenses with a nearsighted prescription simply shrink your world down to the size of your reduced visual field.

Conventional vision care typically does not address the underlying causes of vision problems. It doesn't help you understand and express the fear or rage that distorted your vision in the first place. The eye doctor simply gives you lenses that cast the world into the shape of your fear, bringing it back into clear focus. Then she says, "We have *corrected* your vision."

After you get your new glasses, you can see the world clearly again—but your unresolved fears are still there, and now they're right back in your face. Your protective blur is gone, and you haven't learned any new way to deal with the fear. The last time you felt this way you started shrinking or distorting your field. Now that process is retriggered to create another protective zone to blur out the scary stuff.

The "protective" or "defensive" role that corrective lenses play is often apparent when people who have worn glasses for many years switch to contact lenses. During the first few days they are often aware of a strong, almost physical, sensation that their eyes are unprotected and defenseless. Without their "eye shield" they may even feel anxious when participating in familiar activites, such as playing ball or operating a sewing machine—which suddenly feel threatening to the eyes.

The process of shrinking the field typically continues for years. It is intensified by the "normal" social environment that most of us learn to adapt to as we grow older. As Gottlieb remarks, "We have come to accept as normal some rather unhealthy conditions. The consequences . . . are just now being recognized. . . . It is only within the last decade that . . . attention has begun to focus on the production of stress-related illnesses, a relationship which Bates pointed out . . . decades ago."[6] He describes how Bates felt that "normal" schooling directly aggravates vision problems:

> When the information in schools is presented in uninteresting, non-relevant ways, when the object of such prolonged attention has no inherent motivating interest, the student must develop a means of controlling the mind and body, compelling each by will to do its master's bidding. Some children develop-

ing under these conditions can endure better than others, but some cannot stand the strain; "thus, the schools become the hotbed not only of myopia but of all other [vision problems]."[7]

Although mental and emotional stress can initiate a contraction of the energy field, this collapse may fluctuate for some time before solidifying into an obvious "physical" symptom. One of the major stressors that often turns an energetic withdrawal into a chronic visual "problem" is the physiological stress of reading in the way we are usually taught to read. Recent studies have linked the onset of myopia with close-up visual tasks, especially reading. Researchers are actually speculating that "children learning to read may be experiencing a mild, slow form of pattern deprivation." These results have moved even the *New York Times* to suggest that "a child who is reading might be encouraged to look up every 15 minutes or so."[8] (Chapter 8 contains more detailed suggestions for stress-free reading.)

Our eyes were simply not designed for a lifestyle that involves staying indoors performing such close-up tasks as reading. Add to that the stress of trying to succeed in school or at work, which requires us to focus our attention and ignore our natural impulses, and the energy field is distorted even more. So, as we grow older, our body, mind, and emotions all begin to assume an increasingly stressed, contracted posture. Eventually we are told that we have progressive myopia, or hyperopia, or astigmatism, and so on. The truth is really that our energy field has been encouraged to continue its defensive pattern, and the initial trigger has never been addressed.

As a developmental optometrist, I have worked with thousands of children. Almost invariably, a child can clearly describe the emotional stressors that precipitated the deterioration of her eyesight. In the case of a very young child, the parents can usually pinpoint a stressful situation that occurred just prior to the child's visual deterioration. I have found that other factors which can affect our vision—such as the stress of reading, an indoor lifestyle, and even physical changes in the eye—are unlikely to have a significant effect on our eyesight unless our energetic and emotional field is contracted. When the field shrinks, we lose sight of our relationship to ourselves and the world.

A healthy field is continuously fluctuating. It may shrink from time to time in response to stress, but it soon expands again. It can't get locked into a state of contraction because when we are open to all experiences, self-healing occurs spontaneously and effortlessly. When we are contracted, on the other hand, it feels as if we have to struggle for every tiny shift. How can we expand our visual and energetic field and prevent it from collapsing again in response to every new stressor? There are many different views of healing, and in our culture we are often encouraged to transform ourselves through mental effort. I've found, however, that real change only comes when we let go of the struggle, when we stop *trying,* and that the greatest key to healing our vision is also the simplest one: expanding our awareness.

The Healing Power of Self-Awareness

Like most people, I was raised to believe that life is a painful struggle. I learned to grab with my eyes instead of allowing the world to gently enter my perception. When I discovered Open Focus, I realized that the harder I looked, the more struggle I was creating. I began to see how my vision was simply a reflection of my overall awareness. I saw that life, like vision, is meant to be absolutely effortless. I realized that I didn't have to struggle to create the life I wanted. In fact, effort just made it more difficult. I started to look for the key to effortlessness, to Open Living.

In my practice I saw many people experience immediate visual remissions by either seeing and expressing forgotten emotional traumas or simply recognizing the possibility that their vision could change. Then there was the instantaneous shift in my own vision after my meditative experience—I wondered how such supposedly "physical" changes could take place so quickly. It occurred to me that the only thing that can shift that quickly is our awareness.

I had heard amazing reports of instantaneous shifts of supposedly fixed physiological conditions. Multiple personalities are a striking example. It's not unusual for different personalities within the same body to exhibit dramatically different physical symptoms, including scars, burn marks, cysts, left- and right-handedness,[9] brainwaves, allergies, lifestyles, memories,[10] and even eye pressure and corneal curvature.[11] Michael Talbot notes that "frequently a medical condition possessed by one personality will mysteriously vanish when another personality takes over."[12] He then recounts some of the more mind-boggling findings about these physical shifts:

> By changing personalities, a multiple who is drunk can instantly become sober. . . .
>
> There are cases of women who have two or three menstrual periods each month because each of their subpersonalities has its own cycle. . . .
>
> Speech pathologist Christy Ludlow has found that the voice pattern of each of a multiple's personalities is different, a feat that requires such a deep physiological change that even the most accomplished actor cannot alter his voice enough to disguise his voice pattern. . . .
>
> One multiple, admitted to a hospital for diabetes, baffled her doctors by showing no symptoms when one of her nondiabetic personalities was in control. . . .
>
> There are accounts of epilepsy coming and going and [even] reports that . . . tumors can appear and disappear.

In regard to vision changes, Talbot reports that "visual acuity can differ, and some multiples have to carry two or three different pairs of eyeglasses to accommodate their alternating personalities. One personality can be color blind and another not, and even eye color can change."

A Chicago optometrist found "remarkable changes" in visual acuity between personalities looking through the same eyes: "One patient needed a correction for nearsightedness nearly four times stronger for one personality than another. When she changed into a 6-year-old, her nearsightedness improved to the point that her original childhood prescription corrected her vision. Her teenage personality required an increase in prescription strength but had better vision than her adult selves."[13]

What could possibly have transformed this patient's vision so instantly? It goes against everything we think we know about the human body, which we believe is relatively fixed—our physical structure is supposed to change only incrementally at best. Although it appears unchanging, doctors know that the body is actually in a constant state of flux and regeneration. The evidence of multiple personalities indicates just how much potential we really have to dramatically change our physical conditions.

Awareness seems to determine which potential the body manifests at any given point—the miraculous shift from diabetic to nondiabetic doesn't actually originate in the body. It is simply the physical manifestation of a shift of awareness, which looks like a miracle to us. As Talbot concludes, "We are deeply attached to the inevitability of things. If we have bad vision, we believe we will have bad vision for life, and if we suffer from diabetes, we do not for a moment think our condition might vanish with a change in mood or thought. But the phenomenon of multiple personality challenges this belief and offers further evidence of just how much our psychological states can affect the body's biology."

Although multiple personalities may offer the most dramatic cases, the ability to shift the physical body with our awareness is actually available to everyone at all times. Every time our worldview shifts, we become a different person.

Healing through awareness is within the potential of every person. Some of us only learn to create healing miracles when we face death or a "fatal" diagnosis—but why wait until then? Vision difficulties can be the challenge that stimulates a healing transformation. As we seek a clearer vision of life, we discover that the eyes are simply extensions of our awareness. We discover that clearing our physical sight is the same as clearing our inner sight.

Human Homeopathy

Western (allopathic) medicine currently offers the most effective treatment for many medical conditions. However, it is based on an oppositional approach to health care—that is, it "fights" disease by treating the patient with the opposite, or whatever will induce the opposite, of the symptoms. For example, if you are in pain, you are given painkillers. If you have a fever, you are given drugs to reduce your temperature. The possibility that the pain or the fever itself may have a valuable role in the healing process has become a theoretical issue.

Homeopathy, on the other hand, heals by working in the same direction as the imbalance, by prescribing the vibrational equivalent of the disease—its motto is "like cures like." Homeopathic remedies consist of incredibly diluted solutions (only a few molecules of the active ingredient may be present) of a substance that would normally cause the symptoms at hand. For instance, a common homeopathic remedy for insect bites is apis mellifica, the irritating ingredient in bee stings.

Following the principle of "like attracts like," I've found that our most intense relationships and experiences seem to be a form of *human homeopathy.* The unresolved fears and hurts of our childhood seem to be repeated well into our adult life. In fact, they often form the core of the major challenges in our life until we learn to heal or resolve them. We seem to repeatedly attract situations and relationships that resonate perfectly with our most vulnerable feelings, despite our resolutions to avoid them.

Our childhood traumas often create feelings of deep vulnerability in a particular area of life. To cope, we learn to block out those uncomfortable feelings. However, blocking them out makes it impossible to heal or transform them, so we continue to shut them out of our awareness, because that is all we know. Since we have never learned to acknowledge and experience our discomfort, we tend to revert to a fixed, defensive script based on a past scenario—we get "triggered" and begin to react blindly. In doing so, we may simply be creating a homeopathic magnet that repeatedly draws the same situations into our life until we really begin to see, feel, and heal them. It seems that the universe will continue to provide the curriculum necessary for the evolution of the species. What we resist persists.

The most painful feelings and issues in our life are usually repeated. We keep stepping in the same emotional hole over and over. You'd think we would learn to avoid it after the first few times.

Instead, we continue to walk into our favorite holes. We continue to spend years resisting exactly what we need in order to cure our "nonexistent incurable disorders."

Since we typically spend many years avoiding those difficult feelings, it can be quite a challenge at first to acknowledge them. However, when we begin to feel them fully, painful, self-defeating emotional patterns actually do begin to shift. Emotional healing seems to take place as we allow ourselves to feel our deepest pain. You could say that this process is like allowing a fever to run its course rather than suppressing it with aspirin.

Whenever a person or event triggers those unresolved issues, we feel upset and uncomfortable. This discomfort is a reminder that there's an area in which we need to do some healing. You can check this out yourself. Think of the last time you felt really uncomfortable. Recall that feeling as vividly as you can. Reexperience it as completely as possible. What happened to trigger that feeling? What was your automatic response? How did you interpret this experience?

Now ask yourself, "Have I ever felt these feelings before?" Try to remember the first time you felt this way.

It is almost never the first time, is it? Like vision problems, our most uncomfortable feelings are chronic. They keep coming back until we realize that the problem isn't outside ourselves, in the other person or the external events. The outside events simply create a resonance, a self-recognition, in our vibrational field. When we accept that what we are feeling is truly within ourselves, then we are really ready to begin the healing process.

Now think back to that painful experience or any other difficult experience with a strong emotional charge. Have those feelings come up again since then? How long did it take before you had those feelings again? Then, no matter what changes you decided to make after the first experience, did you eventually get into another situation that felt similar?

Usually, before you know it, you become involved in another experience with the same feeling. This cycle can continue indefinitely. How can we learn to shift out of those blocked places?

Sometimes it seems that the harder we try, the more stuck we feel. But there is a remedy: awareness. Full awareness means that our energy field, our feelings, and all our senses are open and receptive. Expanding our awareness is perhaps the most important step in deeply changing our vision of how we see the world. There is really nothing else to do, because awareness itself is curative.

Awareness Is Being Here Now

What is full awareness and how do we become more aware? Awareness is simply a matter of experiencing every moment of life as fully as possible. Greater awareness does not happen when we try to pay close attention—that effort actually requires a narrowing of one's focus. True awareness is an expansive, effortless process.

Humans have developed a variety of wonderful tricks to avoid being "in the moment." Eastern gurus say that the majority of our mental and physical activities arise from the urge to distract ourselves from our awareness rather than out of any truly purposeful need. I've found that the desire to avoid seeing life fully (and therefore feeling life fully) is also the fundamental origin of vision problems. Most people become bored, anxious, or uncomfortable when they have to sit quietly for even a few minutes—as happened to me when I removed my glasses. Those disconcerting feelings are why we continually seek distractions, and why the Eastern spiritual traditions place so much emphasis on meditation.

Meditation is simply a means of observing our consciousness, usually by fully attending to one thing, such as the breath or a sacred sound, a mantra. Meditation is a very powerful tool for enhancing present moment awareness, and has a cumulative effect when practiced regularly. A feeling of alert and centered attention begins to permeate our being.

There are many ways to access a meditative state. As we have seen, Open Focus (nonjudgmental seeing) can be a form of meditation, a way to become fully present. The next time you're feeling stressed or anxious, try taking a short break to practice Open Focus (as described in Chapter 4). With practice, you'll even be able to stay in Open Focus while going about many of your daily activities. Although the practice of meditation-in-action may sound contradictory, a state of full awareness while acting "in the world" is the ultimate goal of most forms of meditation, and will naturally develop as you meditate regularly.

You don't have to meditate for thirty years to reap the benefits of greater awareness. Every time you practice Open Focus or simply bring your attention back to the present, your energy field and your vision will expand a little bit. Remember that the field usually collapses through a process of alternating expansion and contraction as we narrow our awareness, and as we expand our awareness, it returns to its full range in the same manner.

At first you may not see any difference, but as you continue to remind yourself to attend to the present, you will begin to perceive increasingly subtle shifts—what I call "just noticeable differences." When do you first notice that you are seeing more clearly? When do you first notice that the temperature has changed? When do you first notice that something feels uncomfortable with your spouse or partner?

This enhanced perception is only the beginning—the next step is to express, to speak out about, whatever you are seeing or feeling. This means directly sharing how you feel, what you need, and so on, with those involved. Communication expands the field and invites the next awareness. In fact, our capacity to open up to the world seems to be directly related to our capacity to express ourselves. The path to expanded awareness begins as we nonjudgmentally notice, feel, and communicate our experience in the moment. It sounds so simple, and yet we have such deeply ingrained habits of avoidance. We have forgotten that every time we suppress a perception or an impulse to speak, we limit our life force a little more.

Some people believe that if they follow their impulses, they will do evil or unhealthy things, so they try to control and judge every move. Those ideas are the result of a fear of life, a lack of trust in your own sacred being. I've found that full awareness spontaneously guides us to the most appropriate response to every situation. Every animal relies on its instincts to survive and thrive. Aren't we also meant to be guided by our instinctive self?

Our capacity for full awareness is based on how attentive we are in the present. When we are analyzing rather than feeling our experience, the clarity, energy, and passion that we bring to life is reduced. We may sometimes wonder why we aren't happy, why our life isn't filled with love and joy. Yet sages tell us that happiness is simply the ability to fully appreciate whatever is happening now. The more present we are, the more satisfaction, joy, and love we can both give and receive.

We have been conditioned to believe that life is a difficult struggle. Sometimes we do have painful or frustrating experiences, but I've found that the intensity of the stress is often related to the degree of resistance to being fully in the present. When we remain present, every sensation flows into the next, just as in the old saying "This too shall pass." However, when we feel contracted, we respond as if every pain is permanent and terminal, a threat to our very survival. This belief requires a great deal of effort, stealing away our life force and diminishing our ability to see. But we *can* learn to let go of our fear of life and see clearly.

To see more clearly, we must allow ourselves to feel the discomfort that we've been blurring out of our lives. In the words of Carl Jung, "Neurosis is always a substitute for legitimate suffering." The way to see through the blur is to look at what is hiding within it. One key to spontaneous healing can be found in whatever is happening in your life right now. It isn't somewhere in the past or in the future.

If the world outside appears unclear, it may simply be a signal that something inside is unclear. We've just forgotten how to read that signal. Since we don't understand the blur, we think it is beyond our control, so we "adjust" our vision with a pair of glasses. In so doing, we miss a powerful opportunity to contact the unresolved issues that created the blur in the first place.

Part Two shows how to put all this into practice and clear your own vision. It includes a variety of approaches and practices that have helped thousands of people see a new vision of reality. This possibility is available to everyone, and the first step is a shift of awareness—the willingness to open up and clearly see what we haven't been attending to in life.

6 Vision Quest

DIANA CROW came to see me for a week of therapy in June 1992. She had worn glasses every day since age ten and had been exploring natural vision improvement for a few months. But she hadn't noticed any change in her vision yet. She was wearing a reduced prescription, but since her "real" prescription was over −8.00, even those weaker lenses were very strong "Coke-bottle" lenses.

During our first session, I sensed that her energetic field was quite contracted; it seemed as if she was taking life very seriously, carrying the weight of the world on her shoulders. She agreed that she had always tried very hard to be perfect. I asked her why she had come for treatment. Was it just to heal her eyesight? No, she said, she was really there for self-integration—to heal the whole self. I responded, "Then let's get to work."

I asked Diana to take off her glasses and read the eye chart. The biggest symbol on it was a twelve-inch "7" on the 20/700 line. A person with 20/20 vision would be able to identify it at seven hundred feet. Diana couldn't identify it at twelve feet. I suggested that she begin to experiment with removing her glasses and only wear them when absolutely necessary. She took her glasses off, and after our session she went for a walk around Aspen, getting used to seeing the world through her blur.

She told me the next day that the longer she walked around, the more she seemed to see. She had even begun to experiment with driving without her glasses, which really surprised me since I wouldn't have recommended that with her present degree of myopia. She found that Open Focus helped her to see clearly while driving, and she would put her glasses back on whenever she needed them. Throughout the week she kept exploring her natural vision, gradually building up her confidence.

A few days later Diana had a real breakthrough. She hadn't been very responsive that morning, until I remarked that we had been talking for two days and she hadn't even mentioned John, her husband of twenty-three years. She broke down as she suddenly realized how much she had been denying about her marriage. For twenty-three years she had successfully hidden from herself the awareness that she had gotten married to escape her family. She hadn't allowed herself to see that her "perfect" marriage was an illusion. Now she couldn't avoid it any longer. She saw the truth—and she wanted a divorce.

Right after that remarkable shift of awareness, I checked her vision again. This time she was able to read a letter about three inches tall from twenty feet away—a little better than 20/80 vision. A person with 20/20 vision would be able to read that letter from a distance of eighty feet—Diana had had quite an improvement over just a few days!

As the week went on, I could see that Diana was feeling more and more confident without her glasses, but I was still surprised when she called me the evening after our last session and said that she had driven the 160 miles back to Denver without her glasses. In fact, she had driven over Independence Pass—a steep, winding passage over the Continental Divide that is a challenging drive no matter *how* good your eyesight is.

(Chapter 9 will discuss the topic of driving without glasses in more detail. Diana emphasizes that this choice was not a spur-of-the-moment decision but the culmination of a long process of self-examination and healing. At the time, she felt confident that she could see clearly enough to drive safely. I would add that improving your vision should only assist you in driving more safely and attentively. I recommend that you always drive responsibly and consult with your vision specialist before changing the prescription that you wear while driving.)

When Diana got home, she told her husband she wanted a divorce. Her life changed dramatically as she faced her fears of living alone for the first time and her sadness over her teenage sons' decision to live with their father. For the next three weeks she did not wear her glasses at all and saw very clearly. She drove everywhere without glasses, even in downtown Denver. Then her extended family began to respond to her decision to divorce John, and self-doubt set in again. She felt alone, threatened, and misunderstood—and began to put her glasses back on.

Now, two years later, Diana has glasses with a prescription of about −4.00—about half the prescription she was originally wearing. She doesn't use them all the time, but she keeps them on a string around her neck and puts them on whenever she needs to. With that prescription she can see distances very clearly. Diana feels strongly that deep-seated fear has been the underlying factor in her vision problems, and that her ongoing effort to heal those fears has been the key to improving her vision.

Diana's story illustrates an important element of the vision improvement process: It's not unusual to have a "miraculous" breakthrough and then find that your vision partially blurs again as the underlying, "hidden" feelings begin to surface for resolution. Remember that healthy vision is always adapting and moving, but when you wear lenses, your eyesight is unnaturally fixed in rigid focus. Your vision may fluctuate rapidly for a while as it seeks a more flexible balance—and these shifts are an indication that the healing process is proceeding normally.

By removing your glasses, you have initiated a far-reaching cycle of expansion and healing. Although it can initially be discouraging when your eyesight seems to take "two steps forward and one step back," if you understand these fluctuations, continue to wear corrective lenses only as necessary, and keep your awareness open, your vision *will* continue to improve.

PART
TWO

Vision of a New Reality

7 Change Your Vision, Change Your Life!

Habit is habit, and not to be flung out of the window,
but coaxed downstairs a step at a time.
—Mark Twain

THIS SECTION is a practical guide to making the shift toward holographic vision. It is directed at people who wear corrective lenses, but the suggestions are equally beneficial for those who don't. If you wear lenses, you'll be removing your visual crutches. If you don't wear lenses, you'll be removing the "blinders" from your inner vision. So even if you have good visual acuity, you may want to check out this section before going on to the rest of the book.

We may know that vision improvement is possible but still have no idea how to create it. Even after I experienced Open Focus and the holographic nature of vision, it took me years of clinical practice to shed my misconceptions about how vision improvement occurs. It took me a long time to understand why some people have immediate, spontaneous visual remissions just from seeing that it is possible, while others experience gradual improvements over a few years, and still others never experience any change at all.

We tend to assume that seeing more clearly requires a physical change in the eye muscles (or the eyeball), which we create by doing eye exercises. However, changing our vision is actually no more than a shift of awareness, and in our habit of *trying hard,* most of us make that shift far more difficult than it needs to be. So all the suggestions in this book are primarily *practices in awareness.* Some of them do involve eye movements, but the awareness with which they are done is the true key to lasting change. The movements themselves only produce a temporary shift.

In fact, even the most practical of these exercises aren't really about healing poor eyesight. Vision improvement is actually *a dynamic process of reawakening your insight,* your inner relationship with the world. Only by experiencing this internal process will you achieve a significant and lasting shift in your external sight. If you've already begun to see a new possibility, if you can feel a shift in your beliefs about vision, then your vision has started to improve, whether you can "see" it yet or not. A more open understanding is already beginning to illuminate aspects of your potential that were previously hidden from you.

The focus will not be on end results, such as reading the eye chart perfectly; instead, it will be on continuously returning your awareness to your own experience. You *will* begin to see better, but that improved visual acuity will simply be one by-product of your process of expanding self-awareness. As your whole life begins to expand and shift before your eyes, you may even forget that the initial purpose was simply to see more clearly!

Are you ready to let go of your old beliefs and consider a new possibility? Are you ready to give up your need to blur out the uncomfortable parts of life? Are you ready to trust the perfection of your natural vision?

The Intention to Change

You can begin to heal your vision by getting in touch with your attitudes and beliefs about vision improvement. If you believe that seeing clearly is a physical function of the shape of the eye, then that belief will be your first obstacle to vision improvement. Because of that belief, you will be likely to dismiss anything you might see without glasses as blur interpretation: "That's just my imagination."

Most of us still have that voice in our heads saying that our hope for better vision is a fantasy. As you remove your glasses, you'll find that from time to time that voice will speak up and cast doubt on your progress. You don't need to struggle with your inner voice or try to force it to change. Simply notice it, hear what it has to say, and realize that it is only one aspect of who you are. You'll soon become aware that there is another aspect deep within your being that *knows* you can shift your vision.

It is also important to become aware of your subconscious attitudes toward seeing clearly. Even when we think we know what we want, we may still be subconsciously sending ourselves mixed messages. So it's good to become aware of any underlying doubts or reservations that might be standing in your way. By feeling any "hidden" resistance to change, you actually open the space for new potential.

Try sitting down in a quiet spot and asking yourself: "How do I really want my vision to change?" Take a few minutes to reflect on this. Look at the question from different perspectives and collect the different answers. Then ask yourself: "How would it feel if all of these changes happened right now? How would my life change if I could see perfectly clearly without lenses?"

Almost every lens-wearer will feel some discomfort when honestly considering this question. After all, it means that your protective barrier will be gone. (This can even be a real physical fear for some people—"Without glasses my eyes feel unprotected.")

What is the essence or source of your discomfort, fear, or anxiety? Can you feel a subconscious resistance to seeing clearly? Ask that part of yourself what it's trying to say or do for you. Listen to its answer without judgment and thank it for its efforts on your behalf. Then you can ask it if it is willing to learn a new way to achieve the same goal (of protecting you, for instance) that would allow you to heal your vision as well. Again, listen without judgment and respond to any fears, frustrations, or objections that are raised.

You can continue this conversation until you feel a shift, a willingness to support change.

A New Kind of Vision Care

Some people, especially those who have worn a strong prescription for many years, will feel the need for a "vision mentor" to keep them on track. (Others will get along just fine on their own, using the guidelines in this book to design their own program, and consulting the appendix and bibliography for additional resources.) Since the natural approach to vision improvement is unfamiliar territory for most people, it can be helpful to have a guide who has traveled down the path before. So how do you go about finding that person?

In the past, you may have turned to your eye doctor with questions about your vision, but your eye doctor will not be able to support you with natural vision improvement unless he is familiar with ideas well beyond the mainstream of the profession. Conventional eye-care professionals are taught that vision improvement is impossible, and I've found that most of them continue to accept that view until they have personal experience otherwise. However, the profession now seems to be on the verge of a major shift as more and more practitioners are beginning to recognize the benefits of the holistic perspective.

An excellent source of support is an optometric specialty known as "behavioral optometry," which focuses on preventive and remedial vision care. In addition to the standard training in general optometry, behavioral optometrists have received postdoctoral training in holistic vision care. The holistic approach includes "relationships between vision and movement, balance, posture, orientation and localization in space, spatial judgments, and perception."[1] Behavioral optometrists will generally prescribe reduced prescriptions to support natural vision improvement.

In addition, the field of natural vision improvement itself is also growing rapidly. More and more people who have experienced visual transformation are offering their services to support others through the process. They come from various backgrounds, including optometry, psychology, and a number of other therapeutic approaches. All of this means that you have a better chance than ever of finding a holistic eye doctor or a natural vision improvement practitioner in your local area. (You can start your search by checking the lists in Appendices B and C.)

As you search for professional support for your vision, remember that the idea is to find someone who will listen to you, share in your experience, and empower you to heal yourself. The doctor-patient relationship is rapidly growing beyond the old roles of one individual who thinks he has a problem and another who thinks she has the solution to that problem. The relationship between doctor and patient must now become a true partnership: two individuals working together toward the goal of (mutual) self-healing.

Other than the small specialty of holistic optometry, the vast majority of vision-care professionals are still either unfamiliar with or opposed to remedial vision care. Ophthalmologists—medical doctors specializing in the eye—seem to be particularly opposed to a nonphysical approach to vision. But eye doctors aren't the "bad guys" in this story—they've been just as brainwashed as we were, and many of them are beginning to see the limits of their professional training. So far, however, the majority continue to rely on their familiar beliefs.

A woman in one of my workshops shared this story: She had worn a strong prescription for myopia for many years. Then she started reading about natural vision improvement and decided to stop wearing her glasses. As a result, her eyesight improved so dramatically that she rarely wore them anymore, except on rare occasions.

One day, however, the frame of her "emergency" glasses broke. Since her eyesight had changed so much, she decided to see an ophthalmologist and get a new prescription. The exam went fine, and when it was over he asked to see her old glasses. She pulled them out of her purse and gave them to him. He seemed puzzled.

"There's some mistake here. These aren't your old glasses."

"Yes, they are."

"No, they can't be. These are much stronger than the prescription that I just measured."

"But they are my glasses. I wore them for years."

"That's impossible. I don't believe it."

He kept insisting that they couldn't be her old glasses, and she kept insisting that they were. Finally he said, "Okay, if these really *are* your old glasses, then there must be something wrong with the prescription that I just gave you. I need to reexamine you."

Because of his insistence, she agreed to let him recheck her eyesight. He went through the entire examination again, very carefully, and came up with the same results. "Okay?" she asked, thinking he would now be satisfied. Instead he responded, "No, this just can't be right. There must be something wrong with my equipment. Let me do it again."

He kept checking her eyes until he couldn't think of anything else that could possibly have gone wrong with the exam. He spent hours rechecking her vision and the results never varied, but he was still stumped. He was unable to even consider the possibility that her eyes really could have improved.

Physician, Heal Thyself

More and more eye doctors are becoming receptive to the possibility of natural vision improvement, and even changing their own vision. Christa Roser is an optometrist in Lancaster, Pennsylvania, who attended one of my seminars in April 1992. At the time, her visual acuity was 20/200. Despite the skepticism of her colleagues, she had been trying to reduce her myopia for years. In mid-1993, she sent me this account of her progress:

> I've been without my glasses for over a year now. The last day I wore them was just before your seminar. This is pretty amazing, considering I'd worn them every day since I was in sixth grade. I only wear glasses now for night driving, and even then only one quarter the strength of my old glasses.
>
> At the time of your seminar I had been battling for six years to reduce my myopia, using all kinds of techniques. During the seminar I first realized that I had been fighting to do what was natural—for the mind/body to heal itself. All I had to do was know this and become aware of the changes in my vision.
>
> My unaided visual acuity is now 20/40 in daylight and 20/50 at night. I have bouts of clear vision and can clear my distance vision at will when I notice it's blurry. When I do, it is not at all like the artificial clarity imposed by lenses; it is more three-dimensional, colorful, and alive—almost beyond description. When I neglect my needs for food and sleep, or am nervous or tense, my acuity drops, but when my mind is clear, at rest, calm, and joyful, my vision is great.
>
> I'm not nearly as afraid as I used to be. My confidence and drive are up, as is my physical strength. My husband has even commented about my improved strength and court awareness

in tennis and racquetball. I even find myself getting angry, a previously little-known emotion, which has been a great spark to make positive changes!

In November 1993, I gave a workshop in Sydney, Australia, that was attended by ten optometrists. The first morning I asked them to participate in an experiment by removing their corrective lenses and leaving them off for the duration of the workshop. They agreed to do this, and also gave me permission to use their real names in this book.

Most of them were skeptical. Although they had a professional interest in my work, many of them doubted that their own vision could actually change. I have found, however, that every prescription lens wearer will experience a measurable improvement in their unaided visual acuity if they simply remove their lenses for a few hours. So I checked their unaided vision that morning (just before they put their lenses away), six hours later at the end of the day, and again the next morning (I rechecked only those who had tested less than 20/25). I checked them in front of Dr. Simon Grbevski, who organized the workshop (and whose vision wasn't tested because he had excellent visual acuity).

What did we do during those twenty-four hours? I didn't teach them any "tricks" to improve their vision. I talked about miracles: how they occur around us all the time; how we are continually creating spontaneous healing. I introduced them to a few simple "eye meditations"—sunning, palming, and the Tibetan Wheel (described in Chapter 8). Here are the results of their vision tests:

	Before	**6 hours later**	**24 hours later**
Hans Peter Abel	20/25	$20/20^{-1}$	not retested
Sue Larter	$20/20^{-1}$	$20/10^{-4}$	not retested
Soo Tan	20/600	20/225	$20/25^{-3}$
Elvira Abel	20/400	20/100	$20/25^{-1}$
Jenny Livanos	20/225	20/180	$20/25^{-1}$
Paul Dickson	$20/160^{-1}$	$20/30^{-2}$	20/20
Alan Baily	$20/20^{-3}$	not retested	not retested
Neil Craddock	20/20	not retested	not retested
James Sleeman	20/30	$20/25^{-4}$	not retested

As you read these results, remember that 20/20 is considered "normal" vision, and that the second number gets higher as your vision deteriorates. For instance, a score of 20/200 means that the symbols that this person can identify from twenty feet away could be identified by a person with 20/20 eyesight from two hundred feet away. The superscript numbers (−1, etc.) indicate the number of letters that were not correctly identified in the last line they could read.

Within twenty-four hours, everyone with less than 20/20 eyesight showed improved vision. The greatest changes—by Jenny, Paul, Elvira, and Soo—would be considered no less than miraculous by the standards of conventional eye care! Originally, Soo Tan could only see the eye chart from the standard distance of twenty feet as clearly as a person with normal vision would see it at six hundred feet, but within twenty-four hours she could see it as clearly as they would see it at twenty-five feet.

These results are amazing, but typical of what has happened every time I have asked a group to try this experiment. The only difference is that *this* group was composed of eye-care professionals who had been thoroughly trained to believe that it was impossible! What happened in those twenty-four hours to create such dramatic changes? They were asked to remove their glasses to discover whether the theories they had learned in school would match their direct experience. Later, they were shown a few simple exercises to relax the eye muscles, which some of them did that evening. That is all.

How did they react to this "impossible" shift? I asked Soo Tan, the doctor who had experienced the greatest improvement, to describe the experience in her own words:

> I am forty-one years old and have worn glasses since I was thirteen. On the first day Jacob talked about the possibility of vision improvement. I was not sure if the same thing could happen to me. It did not seem possible at all. As an optometrist, with a career based on giving people glasses to help them, I was not even sure if I wanted that to happen.
>
> That morning our vision was measured and my visual acuity in both eyes was 20/600. I put my glasses away for the rest of

the day. At 4:30 P.M., Jacob measured my vision again, and it was 20/225. I wasn't that excited about it—the improvement was not great enough to move me yet. I drove home wearing a weaker correction than I usually wear, and I could see quite well. That evening I discussed the lecture with my husband, who expressed disbelief and asked, "How are you going to sell glasses?" I was concerned that his attitude would discourage me from continuing to try this approach.

When I drove to the workshop the next morning I decided not to wear any glasses at all. It was quiet on the road because it was Sunday. I did peep through the weaker glasses twice to check the road signs. I was very excited about being able to drive without my glasses. When I got there, Jacob checked my vision again, and I was able to read the 20/25 line with only three errors! The numbers seemed to be doubled and blurry one moment and then suddenly clear the next. It was unbelievable! I was so shocked that I cried for ten minutes.

After I returned to the United States, Dr. Tan wrote to tell me that she had never gone back to her old prescription. She was still having flashes of clear vision, and her "baseline" acuity was slowly improving, fluctuating between 20/200 and 20/20. When her eyes needed a little help, she would put on a prescription of −1.75—less than half as strong as her original lenses.

8 Take Off Your Glasses and See!

You must do the thing you think you cannot do.
—Eleanor Roosevelt

WHEN I FIRST began practicing vision improvement twenty years ago, I just used eye exercises, because I thought exercises created clearer vision. Yet this approach rarely seemed to have a lasting effect. People would start out really excited, and would practice their program faithfully for a week or two. They would see an improvement in their vision, sometimes subtle, sometimes striking. Then they would stop doing the exercises and the changes would stop. If they returned to wearing their old prescription, the improvement might even reverse itself.

Then I started seeing more and more people experiencing immediate, lasting vision improvements without doing any exercises at all! I began to wonder whether the change was caused by the exercises or by some other factor. Since then, I have confirmed my suspicion that the shift to a new way of seeing is not physical; it has more to do with the willingness to accept an expanded vision of life. If you are just doing the eye exercises, without being willing to transform how you see the world, the exercises are unlikely to have a significant, lasting effect on your vision. If you understand that you are truly on a "vision quest," then you'll be on a path toward profound healing and transformation on all levels of your awareness—and the exercises can be tools that support your progress.

Seeing the Flash

Here's an example of how an effortless shift of awareness can spontaneously transform eyesight. I was working with a client who was unable to make out the letters on the eye chart—he was trying very hard, but he still couldn't see them. I suggested, "Close your eyes and breathe in gently." He began to gasp for air, with his shoulders raised and his chest pushed out. Then he held his breath, opened his eyes, and tried to read the chart again. He couldn't see any better. Like all of us, his problem wasn't that he didn't know how to see; it was that he didn't know how to live.

I said, "Close your eyes and visualize that your body is a balloon very slowly filling with air. When it's full, allow the balloon to gently deflate, at its own speed. Then, very gently and softly, with no intention at all, open your eyes and allow the world to see you." When he did this, he could immediately see more clearly. By the time he had practiced this gentle breathing for a few minutes, his vision had improved from just under 20/200 to 20/40. All he had done was adjust his relationship to the world.

Afterward he commented, "You know, for a moment there, when I first opened my eyes, everything was crystal clear, and then it got all fuzzy again." This reminded me that I had had the same experience when I first started taking off my glasses. Since then, I've noticed that there is an instant in which we all see clearly every time we open our eyes. Healing our vision is simply allowing that instant to get longer and longer, until it becomes our normal way of seeing.

In that first instant, we aren't yet *trying* to see; our mental and emotional conditioning takes a moment to move into place. We are fully transparent, without effort or expectations, and our perceptive field reflects that openness. My client saw the world clearly in that moment because *he* was clear. Although we all experience that unclouded vision automatically when we first open our eyes, for most of us that flash is so brief that our awareness no longer registers it. Our vision seems to instantly shift into its "normal" distortion as our self-limiting beliefs snap into place.

Most people can easily experience that clarity by simply bringing their attention to it. I'll guide you through a way to practice that attention, but remember that the harder you try, the less you'll see—so go easy on yourself! (To get the best results with the practices in this book, tape-record the directions and play them back to yourself. Or even better, have a friend read them to you and make sure that you keep breathing easily and don't strain. Then you can switch places.)

Start by taking off your glasses or contacts and finding a comfortable, relaxed position. Take a minute to bring your attention within yourself. Allow it to wander through your body, becoming aware of any tension or discomfort. As you do this, allow your breathing to become soft and gentle. You may want to use the balloon image: Imagine that you are very slowly and softly blowing up your balloon-body with air. When you feel full, don't collapse your breath or strain at the fullness—just allow the flow of air to reverse itself, still without any effort or straining.

Continue breathing and allow your eyes to close gently. Bring your attention to your eye sockets and notice any feelings of "holding on" or "grabbing" there. Don't try to make it better, just spend a few moments feeling that tension. Imagine that you are breathing in and out through your eyes. As you breathe, allow a feeling of softness and gentleness to gradually seep into your eye sockets. Notice how the grabbing begins to shift by itself. Enjoy this process for a while.

Then, as you exhale, very gently and slowly allow your eyes to open. As you open them, don't look at anything, or worry about whether you will see clearly. Allow the room to look at you. When your eyes are open, start to inhale, and allow them to effortlessly close again. There's no need to squint; keep your eye muscles very soft and easy the whole time. Continue to gently open and close your eyes along with your breath.

Now notice a kind of movement or wobble that seems to occur just as your eyes are opening. As you continue to open and close your eyes, allow your attention to become fascinated by that wobble. Notice how it almost looks as if the room is moving or shifting as your eyes first open. Notice how your vision in that instant is different from the stabilized state just after it—not better or worse, just different.

Continue doing this for a few minutes, until you get bored or find that you're beginning to strain at it. Once you get the hang of it, you can practice it every day. It may seem simple, but the challenge is to use as little effort as possible and remain far more open and effortless than usual. The more you practice, the more you'll start having spontaneous flashes of perfectly clear vision, not only during the exercise but at any time of day. Yet you won't be able to see those flashes unless you take the most important step in strengthening your vision: removing the crutches from your eyes!

Removing Your Blinders

Recognizing that change is possible and removing your lenses (or reducing your prescription) are the most important steps you can take to see better. In my workshops, I see repeatedly that just taking these two steps is all most people need to significantly improve their vision. Typically, every participant with less than optimal vision will have measurable improvement within hours just by removing his glasses and considering the possibility of change.

To experience this for yourself, try this experiment. First, remove your prescription lenses and look around you. How well are you seeing now? The world looks pretty blurry, right? Remember the eye chart you removed from the book and put up on your wall (pages 111 to 114)? Use that chart to recheck your vision now, right after removing your lenses. (If you've already started leaving your lenses off, don't put them back on. In that case you may not notice such striking results from this exercise, since your vision has already begun to readjust itself.) You don't need to calculate the exact level of your visual acuity; simply put the chart up on the wall and determine the smallest line that you can see clearly, without straining or squinting.

Afterward, do not put your lenses back on! Go outside and take a leisurely twenty-minute walk, leaving your lenses at home or in your pocket the entire time. As you walk, breathe fully and don't strain to see the world. Just notice whatever you are seeing, without the judgments of "It's blurry" or "It's clear."

When you return, check your vision again the same way you did before.

Most people who try this experiment find a noticeable improvement in their acuity. How can simply removing your glasses clear your vision? Taking off those crutches allows your eyes to readjust to seeing on their own. The longer you keep your glasses off, the more you will notice the constant fluctuation of your eyesight. Sometimes you may have flashes of perfectly clear vision; at other times your vision may appear to be worse. This dynamic fluctuation is a sign that a healthy visual function is reasserting itself after being locked in a rigid focus for many years. Unlocking that focus is the first step toward reclaiming your naturally clear vision.

In late 1993, I visited my friends Nada and Simon Grbevski in Australia (Simon was hosting the optometrists' workshop described in the previous chapter). Nada had worn a strong prescription for years, and I suggested that we do a little experiment. She removed her glasses and less than fifteen minutes later read the 20/40 line on the eye chart with only one error. Then we took a walk. She was so overwhelmed by the clarity of her vision that she had to look away, saying "I had been trying to make out the words on a distant billboard. [Finally] it became crystal clear! I was startled and overcome with a feeling of both panic and excitement. The feeling of panic was so powerful that I forced myself to look away and return to my safe home of blur."

Nada returned to wearing her glasses, and the next day I checked her vision again, but now she could see only 20/400! The same letters that she could see from four hundred feet the day before she could now only see from forty feet. When she put her glasses back on for just one day, we discovered that her vision had decreased significantly. A few months later she wrote to tell me that this experience had made such a big impression on her that she never did put her glasses back on. She said that her visual acuity had returned to 20/40 and that she has learned to clear her vision completely as needed.

If you are now wearing a strong prescription, I suggest that you get a weaker prescription—"training lenses"—to wean yourself away from your maximum correction and allow your natural vision to return. (Appendix B contains a list of optometrists who are willing to prescribe lenses with a weaker prescription.) Removing powerful lenses all at once can be like quitting any addiction "cold turkey." After wearing them for years, you may only be able to keep them off for short periods at first. You may become anxious or uncomfortable without your lenses, or feel that you are unable to see clearly enough to drive or work, but every time you remove them you begin to access your ability to see more clearly. Every time you put your lenses back on, however, your vision starts to contract again, and the stronger the correction, the more it will be forced to contract.

You'll want lenses for working or driving that support your continually improving vision—the minimum safe correction required for those activities, rather than the maximum. You may be surprised to discover how much you can reduce your prescription and still see well enough to drive safely and work effectively.

If you have both contacts and glasses, you may want to consider only wearing your glasses (with a weaker prescription) for a while. You're going to be noticing that you don't need your lenses nearly as much as you thought you did, and it's much easier to take glasses on and off, as needed, than contacts. It can also be helpful to get an eyeglass chain to wear around your neck. This makes it even easier to put your glasses on only when you need them.

No matter how "weak" your eyesight is, you are very likely wearing your prescription more than you really need to. Most people find that there are very few activities that really require the full prescription that eye doctors are trained to provide, because those prescriptions are based on our worst-case visual need. Do we really need the same prescription to drive in a rainstorm at night as we do to read a book outside on a sunny day? Absolutely not! So if you're myopic, get in the habit of always taking off your glasses for eating, reading, and other close-up work. When your eyes do need some support, use your weaker lenses as much as you can. Reserve your strongest prescription for the most visually demanding activities, such as night driving.

Using the same long-distance focus for all activities teaches the eyes to suppress their ability to adapt to every new situation. Since "what you don't use, you lose," it's important to be patient as your eyes recover the natural functions that haven't been used in years. Whenever you're trying to see something that appears blurry, take a few unhurried moments to pause, breathe, and blink before you say, "I can't see it." Give your eyes the chance to respond, to remember how to see.

When you take that moment to allow your eyes to adjust, you'll be surprised at how well you can see without your glasses. You'll see that most of the time, when you reach for your glasses, it's because you're feeling uncomfortable or anxious, not because you really need them. For instance, most people find that they don't really need their glasses for such common activities as eating, exercising, reading, writing, having a conversation, shopping, cooking, doing the dishes, or going to the bathroom. When you don't need them, take them off! The longer you can keep them off, the more activities you'll discover that you don't need them for. Wearing glasses is like any other habit: The more you do it, the harder it is not to do it; the less you do it, the easier it is not to do it.

Vision Meditations

Now we will look at some practical suggestions to support your vision improvement process. Again, remember that the exercises do not create the improvement, they merely assist its progress. The state of mind in which you do them is actually more important than any of the physical movements. I like to call these practices "vision meditations," rather than "eye exercises," to keep this meditative state in mind.

Most people find that it is fun and easy to add a few vision meditations to their daily routine. The simplest place to start is to just ask yourself as you go through your day, "What am I seeing *now*?"

Breath Awareness

Breath is the flow of our life force, our link to the web of life. The way we draw air into our lungs is a mirror of the way we take life into our awareness. When we feel stressed, we automatically suppress or hold our breath. When we feel relaxed, our breath flows freely, reducing stress and enhancing self-integration. Since effortless, relaxed breathing cannot occur in a contracted field, we can even use the breath to relax and expand the energetic and visual fields.

Most Westerners don't think too much about breathing. We assume that it is simply a way to pump air in and out of the lungs. The Indian yogis, however, knew that the breath is a direct reflection of our awareness. Bija Bennett, a yoga therapist, has written a wonderful book called *Breathing into Life,* about using the breath to enhance awareness and healing. She begins by describing "the power of the breath":

> It's true that every emotion, physical condition, resistance, disturbance, or tension you have is connected to your breath.
>
> Do you ever notice that you are holding your breath? Remember what you do when you are afraid, tense, or worrying about something? Or how your breath is when you've been sitting at your desk all day?
>
> It's the breath that is carrying the message.
>
> The breath can be your best friend. It can be a tool to balance, release, and free your mind and body. It can bring you strength and courage. It can calm you down or give you energy.
>
> Breathing is an art.
>
> But you don't need to be taught *how* to breathe.
>
> *Breathing needs not to be taught, but liberated.*
>
> Gentle, conscious, flowing, moving—
> *the power of the breath.*[1]

Since breath awareness is the doorway to the meditative state, it is the first step in all the exercises and suggestions in this book. You can begin tuning in to your breath at any time.

Remove your lenses and take a moment to notice your breath. The air comes in—and where does it go? Does it go into your chest? Does it go into your abdomen? Does it go anywhere else? Does it feel blocked or frozen anywhere in your body? Does it feel shallow or deep, fast or slow, easy or difficult? Are you aware of any effort in the intake or release of your breath?

Most of us limit our breath to the upper chest, which reflects a lot of holding and contraction. Most yogis practice some form of belly breathing, but a full breath doesn't even stop in the belly, and we can all learn to easily and spontaneously extend the range of our breath.

Bring your attention to your breath. Begin to breathe gently and effortlessly. Allow your breath to move freely. Before long you may notice that your breath seems to deepen. Just notice that and keep your attention on your breath. After a few more deep breaths, you may start to feel your shoulders or your back relaxing, as if they were releasing a heavy burden. Then your lower body may open up, as your breath effortlessly moves all the way through your torso and down your legs.

Whenever you notice that your mind has gone elsewhere, return your attention to the breath.

While you were breathing, did you find yourself thinking about something else? Did your mind suddenly go off and running? Wandering is normal for the mind, just as it is for the eyes, but when we are thinking, we generally aren't fully aware. Whenever you notice yourself thinking, gently bring your attention back to your breath. After a while you'll notice that your mind is getting quieter and quieter.

Breath awareness is not about trying to relax or to keep the mind quiet or any other activity. It is simply a practice of being fully aware. As you center your attention on whatever your breath wants to do, you open up and allow more and more vital energy to flow into your mind/body.

If you lie down and continue to gently practice breath awareness, you may notice how the vital energy seems to fill you up right down to your toes. Check in then and observe how open and relaxed you feel: This is the feeling of an open energy field. It is how we are meant to live and see all the time. Now open your eyes for a moment and notice your vision, remaining in that easy, relaxed state of aware breathing. You may or may not notice any difference in your eyesight at this point, so just welcome whatever you see, without judgment.

Breath awareness is so important. You might want to put up little signs that say, "Breathe!" all around you—on your bathroom door, on your refrigerator, on your car dashboard—to keep reminding you of the power of the breath.

Remember to Blink

We normally take blinking for granted. It just happens automatically, right? Not necessarily. Dr. William Bates was the first person to point out that chronic vision problems seem to be invariably associated with an unblinking stare. As Aldous Huxley explains,

> Eyes in a condition of dynamic relaxation blink often and easily. But where there is strain, blinking tends to occur less frequently and the eyelids work tensely. . . . The inhibition of movement . . . is carried over, not only to the eyes, but to their lids as well. A person who stares closes the eyelids only at long intervals. . . .
>
> But so long as the eyelids are kept tense and relatively immobile, the eyes themselves will remain tense and relatively immobile. . . . Consequently, anyone who wishes to acquire the art of seeing well must cultivate the habit of frequent and effortless blinking.[2]

Although we are usually unaware that we are staring, with a little attention we can learn to sense when we are keeping our eyelids fixed open. Staring is especially common when we feel stressed. Whenever you feel tense or tired, or whenever you remove your glasses, take a few rapid, soft blinks—"butterfly kisses." Every once in a while, squeeze your eyelids tightly closed for a second—you can do that instead of rubbing your eyes, for instance.

A habit of frequent blinking throughout the day will help keep your eyes soft and relaxed. Anytime you notice that your vision feels tense or blurry, a few gentle blinks can work wonders—especially in combination with Open Focus (pages 44 and 102).

Tracing

William Bates was the first person to notice that consciously mimicking the continuous movement of healthy eyes can significantly sharpen visual clarity and reform the habit of staring. He suggested tracing the outlines of everything around us:

> Remove your lenses and look up from the page. Notice what your eyes are doing—are you holding your eyes open, trying to see everything all at once? Now close your eyes and visualize what you have just seen. Does your inner picture feel complete? Do your inner eyes feel clear, or do they feel somehow "out of touch" with your vision?
>
> Open your eyes again. Allow yourself to blink and take a few deep breaths. Notice that as your eyes begin to relax, they want to *move* rather than stare. Allow them to be drawn toward the most prominent shape or object. Select one point along its edge or boundary. Begin to move your eyes along that edge, in little increments. Don't try to see the object as a whole. Simply trace the outlines of all its boundaries and prominent features, one point at a time.
>
> Now close your eyes and again visualize what you have just seen. Does your inner picture seem to be more complete, more accurate than before? Do you feel more "in touch with" what you have seen?

I've been asked, "Doesn't 'tracing' contradict the whole idea of Open Focus? After all, in Open Focus we see the whole scene with equal clarity, and now you're suggesting that we do just the opposite!" The link between these two practices is continuous eye movement. In Open Focus we allow it to occur spontaneously, and in tracing we do it consciously, but in both cases the eyes are in constant motion. Our habitually stressed way of seeing, on the other hand, actually fixes the eyes in place, in an unblinking stare.

Huxley has a very interesting suggestion about tracing, which he calls "shifting":

> Persons with defective sight tend to do some of the intensest and most rigid staring when conversing with their fellow humans. Faces are very important to us, since it is by observing their changes of expression that we acquire much of our most valuable information . . . [so we] stare harder than usual. The result is discomfort and embarrassment for the persons stared at, and poorer vision for the starer. . . . [So] do not

stare at faces, in the vain hope of seeing every part of them as clearly as every other part. Instead, shift the [gaze] rapidly over the face . . . from eye to eye, from ear to ear, from mouth to forehead. You will see the details of the face and its expression more clearly, and to the person you are looking at, you will seem to be merely looking in a relaxed and easy way, with eyes to which your rapid, small-scale shifting imparts the brilliancy and sparkle of mobility.[3]

Even a few minutes of tracing can powerfully improve the clarity of your vision. To really *see* this, you might set aside twenty minutes at the beginning of each day to play with Open Focus, blinking, breath awareness, tracing, and swinging (the next eye meditation). You'll be amazed at how quickly your vision will clear once you remove your lenses and your eyes start to move again!

Swinging

Swinging is another fun practice that can help to relax your entire body and also reprogram the naturally smooth, flowing movement of the eyes:

Remove your lenses and stand in a comfortable position with your feet about shoulder-width apart and your arms hanging freely at your sides. Take a full breath, allow your shoulders to relax, and begin to gently twist your body to the left. Notice that as you turn left, your weight shifts onto your left foot, and your right heel is raised off the floor. When you reach the limit of your range of motion, begin to move at the same even pace toward the right. Notice the relaxation occurring along your spine.

As you move, look softly and imagine that your eyes are a brush painting a sweeping horizontal stroke across your field of vision. Notice that the world appears to flow past you in the opposite direction.

If you aren't seeing this motion, blink, breathe, and look effortlessly into the air as you move from side to side. Don't try to *focus on* or *look at* any of the moving objects.

Begin with ten to fifteen swings and gradually increase to fifty. Allow yourself to be fully aware of each moment as you swing from side to side.

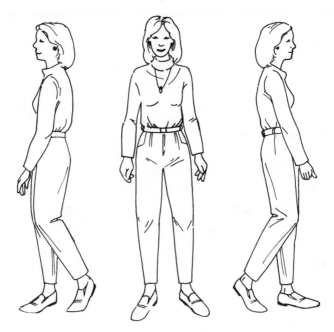

Swinging Procedure

Open Focus

This is a good place to review the Open Focus meditation, because you'll be using it a lot as you remove your glasses. Open Focus reminds us that the less we *try to see,* the more our vision will effortlessly become clear. Practicing Open Focus as often as possible throughout the day will help keep your vision open and relaxed.

> Remove your glasses or contacts, and look up at your surroundings. Locate any object that you can see relatively clearly and experiment with your focus. Focus on it really hard, and then look at it more softly. Notice that the more intensely you focus, the less of everything else you can see. Notice that when you focus really hard, your entire peripheral vision closes down.
>
> Now look at the same object without focusing or staring rigidly. Become aware of your breath. Allow your visual focus to soften and expand until you can see not only the first object but everything around it with equally Open Focus. Notice how

you can expand this farther to see everything in your visual field, still without focusing or fixing your gaze. Everything you see looks equally important, and your eyes are in continuous, spontaneous movement.

Palming

Developed in the 1920s by Dr. William Bates, palming is an excellent way to refresh your body/mind while improving your vision. It is also a wonderfully simple way to take time to nurture yourself. Every time you palm, your field opens and the life force can flow effortlessly through you. If you palm regularly, you'll feel more centered and less stressed.

Palming can be done at any time, and for as long and as often as you like. I suggest that you palm before and after all of the other eye meditations so as to allow your eyes to rest after each activity. Here's how to get started:

> Move your chair to a desk or table on which you have built a stack of books that is high enough for you to comfortably rest your elbows on it without hunching over. This will ensure that your neck, back, and shoulders are relaxed and supported. Get into a comfortable sitting position with your feet flat on the floor.
>
> Warm your hands by briskly rubbing them together. Resting your elbows on the books, close your eyes and gently move your cupped hands toward your face. As your hands approach your face, move in slowly—don't startle yourself.
>
> Allow your hands to follow a natural line of movement up to your eyes. Allow one hand to fall over the other, as illustrated on the following page, so that the center of each palm is directly over each eye (but not touching the eye), and the heels of the hands are resting on the cheekbones. Fold your hands gently around your nose, allowing the breathing cavity to remain open. Don't put any pressure on your nose, your cheeks, or your eyes.
>
> Bring your attention to your breath, breathing gently and effortlessly. Notice how the total darkness soothes your eyes and allows your entire mind/body to relax. If you notice yourself thinking, gently bring your attention back to your breath.

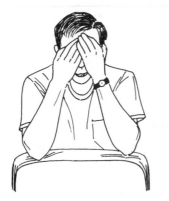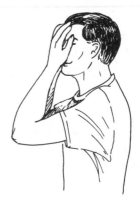

Palming Procedure

When you feel complete, slowly put your hands down and open your eyes. Before jumping back into your day, take a few moments to appreciate how gentle you feel. Notice that your vision is sharper and brighter than before. See if you can maintain this soft feeling as you return to your activities.

I suggest that you begin by doing twenty one-minute sessions of palming daily, but you can always increase the length of any session as needed. You can do palming and breath awareness in the morning, to awaken gently, and at bedtime, to help you fall asleep. If you palm while lying in bed, I suggest that you place a few pillows under your elbows to support your arms.

Sunning

Sunning was also developed by Dr. Bates, who used it as an eyesight improvement technique, but it does far more than sharpen the vision. Our body is actually a living photoelectric cell that is stimulated and regulated by light energy from the sun. Good health requires daily doses of sunlight, and yet few of us are getting our minimum daily requirement of light energy. In fact, on the average, Americans spend only 3 percent of their lives outdoors.

You know what jet lag feels like? Well, many people are chronically jet lagged and haven't even been near an airplane. Most of us use nonprescription stimulants and depressants (like caffeine, sugar, alcohol, and nicotine) every day. Over time, these substances alter our biological clocks so that they fall out of sync with the natural cycles regulated by light and darkness. Sunning twice a day, at sunrise and sunset, can resynchronize you with Nature's rhythms.

> Begin by taking off your lenses and going outside into direct sunlight. (If it's warm enough, take off your shoes and stand in your bare feet on the earth.) Close your eyes, bend your knees slightly, and fully face the sun. Bring your attention to your breath. Begin to turn your head very slowly to the right, letting the sun bathe your closed eyelids. When you have turned your head all the way to the right, very slowly turn back to the left. Continue moving your head all the way to the left. Keep your eyes softly closed and your attention on your breath. Do this slow back-and-forth movement a few times.
>
> Then repeat the same movement vertically: Move your head down to your chest and then move it all the way up and back, allowing the sunlight to stimulate the midline of your face and scalp. Do this a few times, very slowly.
>
> Afterward, don't open your eyes right away. Palm and breathe until any afterimages disappear.

This only takes a few minutes and is a nice morning and evening meditation. A regular practice of sunning is especially important for light-sensitive people. As our eyes absorb direct sunlight through closed lids, they regain their ability to adapt to strong light without straining. Therefore sunning is very helpful in weaning ourselves from dependence on sunglasses and reducing light sensitivity in general.

You can practice sunning anytime during daylight, but it is easiest in the early morning and late afternoon, when the sun is low in the sky and you don't have to strain your neck. You can also use this technique on a cloudy or rainy day. Even then, the sunlight filtered through the clouds is much brighter than artificial light indoors. If it's really bad weather, you can sun from a screened porch, but don't try sunning from behind a window or windshield, as the glass shuts out some of the natural light spectrum.

Some people I have worked with live in high-rise apartments or on a mountainside where sunlight is rare. I have suggested that they get a clip-on lamp with a 150-watt floodlight. This can be used as the sun if you stand three feet away from it. However, always go

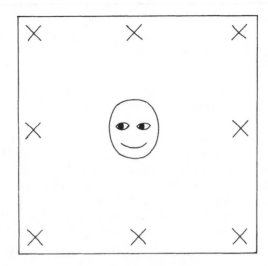

Position of Stickers on Window for Passive Seeing
Place the stickers on the spots marked *X*. The circle in the middle of the square shows the ideal head position.

outside if at all possible, because there really is no substitute for natural sunlight.

Passive Seeing

Here's an interesting set of meditations that help us to dissolve our hard focus and see effortlessly (I'd like to thank Ray Gottlieb for introducing them to me). You can do this for about ten minutes a day. Begin slowly, and breathe and blink fluidly throughout the exercise. Be very easy with yourself. Doing this exercise with a soft, gentle awareness will lead you into a meditative state in which effortless vision can occur:

> Place a chair approximately five feet from a full-size window or a sliding-glass door. Sit in the chair and adjust its height until your head is about level with the middle of the window. Draw a large *X* on eight pieces of colored paper or Post-it stickers, and attach them to each corner and midpoint of the window (see the illustration above).

Sit in the chair and take a few gentle breaths. Now, using the Post-it stickers as markers, begin to move your eyes horizontally back and forth between the two markers at eye level. Move your eyes back and forth rhythmically about once per second.

Move your eyes horizontally (center right to center left), then vertically (center top to center bottom), then diagonally (corner to corner, both ways). As your eyes move, continuously breathe, blink, and be aware of any holding or tension in your body.

Allow your eyes to move easily and rhythmically back and forth—and they will soon begin to move for you. Don't "try" to relax if you still feel tension, just let the breath do it for you.

This exercise has you doing a very simple task—much simpler than reading, for instance. Yet what happened to your breath as you were moving your eyes back and forth? If you're not sure, try it again.

Most people either stop breathing or try to synchronize their breathing to the beat. Paying attention does not require you to synchronize your breath to the rhythm of the activity. It's only when you are trying to stay in control that you stop breathing spontaneously. This meditation helps you to become aware of and to release that holding response.

Once you are familiar with the basic procedure, you can make your own variations and practice it anywhere. You might do it anytime you have to wait or stand in a line, for instance—just remember to breathe, blink, and be aware of tension. Here are some more variations to play with:

1. Move your chair closer or farther away from the targets.

2. If you have a metronome, use it to vary the speed of the movements, always maintaining a meditative state. Gradually develop faster or slower speeds. Change the speed each time only when you are able to do it effortlessly at the current speed.

3. Place one target (such as a pocket calendar) at reading distance and eye level, and pick another one outside the

window. Allow your eyes to move from the near target to the one farther away. As your eyes move back and forth, notice if the near and far targets are in focus. If your eyes are working together, the target you are focused on will appear single while the other will appear double. If you are not seeing this, continue the meditation until you are.

Tibetan Wheel

When the eyes and mind are relaxed, our eye muscles are flexible and instantly adjust to our every visual need; but just as overdependence on crutches weakens leg muscles by removing their normal activity, so overdependence on glasses weakens the eye muscles. Unused muscles not only become inflexible, they actually weaken the entire system as the body adapts to the artificial limits on its normal functioning. The Tibetan Wheel is a way to help underused eye muscles regain their former flexibility.

Our eye movements allow us to access the information stored in our memory banks, but when we restrict those eye movements in response to stress, we lose some of that spontaneous ability. The Tibetan Wheel can help to relax the eye muscles so that those files become more accessible with less effort. It stretches and tones all the eye's muscles, including those that may not be used regularly. For best results, do this exercise twice every day, once in the early morning (before breakfast) and once in the early evening (before dinner).

Photocopy and enlarge (to about 8½" by 11") the illustration of the Tibetan Wheel. Attach it to any convenient wall, placing the central spot level with the tip of your nose. Take off your glasses or contacts, and stand directly in front of the chart at a visually comfortable distance. You will start farther away and move closer as your eye muscles become more flexible. The easiest way to do this is to mark your position on the floor with a piece of tape, and move it forward an inch every week.

Turn your attention to your breath. When you feel ready, find a point anywhere on the outer edge of the wheel and very

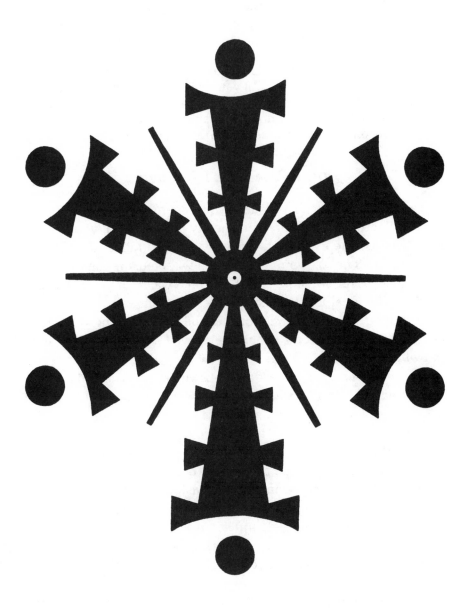

Tibetan Wheel

slowly move your eyes clockwise, outlining the outer edge of each arm, including the black circles, until you return to the original point. Keep your head still and let your eyes move. Do not push or strain, and be sure to blink and breathe throughout the exercise. (If it becomes uncomfortable, stop and palm, and continue later.)

Palm for one minute, then repeat counterclockwise. When you are done, palm again until your eyes feel soft and relaxed.

As always, breath awareness is critical. This meditation has very little value if it isn't done with an open breath. Otherwise it just becomes another muscular strain on the eyes.

How to Use Your Eye Chart

You can use the eye chart to help you become more aware of the constant fluctuation of your visual acuity and range. (If you haven't yet assembled the eye chart, you may wish to follow the instructions on page 3 now): From now on you will be using the eye chart on a regular basis, so find a spot for it on a wall that you see every morning. The ideal location is right across from your bed, so it is the first thing you see in the morning and the last thing you see at night. For the best effect it should be at eye level and ten feet or so from where you sit up in bed.

Don't think of this as "checking" your vision every morning—this is not an acuity test. It is simply an easy way to observe the natural fluctuations of your vision; it's really an open-eye meditation. You can practice Open Focus looking toward the eye chart, or just relax and trace the outlines of whatever you are seeing—or just be aware of your breath and continue to blink naturally. Soon you may begin to notice how the fluctuations in your vision are related to factors such as your state of mind, the time of day, the amount of light, weather conditions, your diet, and so on.

How do you feel when you are seeing clearly? How do you feel when all you see is blur? Can you feel how your energy field is fluctuating as your vision shifts?

If you do this regularly, you'll become familiar with your visual fluctuations. You'll see how your eyesight seems to mirror your inner state. When we feel joyful, we usually see with greater clarity

$$\frac{20}{400}$$

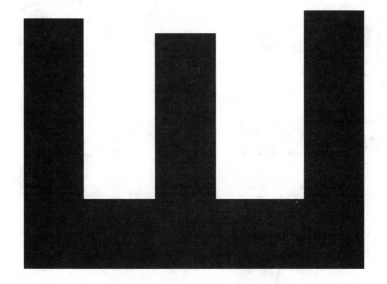

$\frac{20}{200}$

$\frac{20}{160}$

K R

L V D

$\frac{20}{125}$ $\frac{20}{100}$ $\frac{20}{80}$ $\frac{20}{70}$

C N D E
H R V K
S K R P
Z H C N
C D

$\frac{20}{60}$	$\frac{20}{50}$	$\frac{20}{40}$	$\frac{20}{30}$	$\frac{20}{25}$	$\frac{20}{20}$	$\frac{20}{16}$
HONSDCV	OKHDNRCS	VHDNKUOSRC	BDCLKZVHSROA	HKGBCANOMPVESR	PKUEOBTVXRMJHCAZDI	DKNTWULJSPXVMRAHCFOYZG

than when we feel depressed or anxious. Wearing corrective lenses tends to maintain or even increase that internal stress. When we decrease our prescription or remove our prescription lenses, it helps to relax every part of the body/mind.

Tips for Good Visual Hygiene

Even after learning to remove your glasses, breathe, and blink, many common activities—reading, watching TV, working at a computer, and wearing sunglasses—can still be stressful to your visual health. For most of us, removing these activities from our daily lives is just not possible, so it can be helpful to simply be more aware of how they are affecting your vision. Here are a few "visual hygiene" tips and suggestions to help you extend your vision quest to these situations.

Use Plus Lenses to Reduce Near-Point Stress

The human eye is primarily designed for distance vision in natural sunlight, not close-up work under artificial light. So most people experience some level of visual strain or fatigue when doing close-up tasks—behavioral optometrists call this "near-point stress." There is much evidence that the epidemic of poor eyesight is directly related to near-point stress. For instance, in a major study of more than 160,000 schoolchildren, it was found that unless preventive measures were taken, by the end of the fifth grade about 80 percent of the schoolchildren developed measurable vision problems.[4] This effect was believed to be the result of several factors, including near-point stress during reading.

Behavioral optometrists have been researching the problem of near-point stress since the 1920s and have discovered a wonderful tool to ease its effects: Plus Lenses. These are very low-powered magnifying lenses, similar to those usually prescribed for farsightedness but much weaker. Although Plus Lenses are not usually used to correct visual acuity, they have been found to have other significant therapeutic effects.

Studies have shown that Plus Lenses reduce physiological stress—blood pressure, respiration rate, pulse rate, and such. This relaxation is probably caused by the subtle diffusion of focus that the lenses create. As soon as you put them on, you are encouraged to look at the world more softly, and your field tends to expand. By reducing stress, Plus Lenses seem to directly affect the contracted field—the underlying source of most vision problems. This may be why they are often effective in reversing the early stages of near-sightedness in children. They seem to act as a wedge that subtly nudges the contracting field back toward openness.

Plus Lenses are helpful for students of all ages, and most people can benefit from wearing them for close-up activities (nearsighted people would simply wear a reduced prescription, which has the same effect as wearing a Plus Lens). However, they are probably most valuable for children with learning difficulties, to enhance their performance in school and prevent future vision problems. They can immediately improve many aspects of the child's behavior and performance, including reading skills, memory, general coordination, and social skills.

How can Plus Lenses improve learning difficulties without any significant effect on visual acuity? Researchers are beginning to see powerful connections between vision problems, learning disabilities, and antisocial behavior (Chapter 15 covers this in more detail). They've discovered that the most common vision problems may actually be unrelated to how clearly we see. Most children classified as nonreaders or juvenile delinquents have 20/20 eyesight, but still have significant vision problems (such as erratic eye movement, poor eye-teaming skills, and difficulty in focusing) that profoundly affect their behavior and ability to learn.

In one study, 96 percent of hard-core juvenile offenders were found to have significant vision problems (although they did *not* have poor visual acuity).[5] After receiving a program of vision therapy, their rearrest rate dropped from about 50 percent to 10 percent and their reading skills improved by four grade levels. In addition, their self-esteem, IQ, and positive values were also enhanced.

Plus Lenses may allow a child who normally has difficulty catching a ball without dropping it to suddenly be able to catch with accuracy. They may allow a child who is a word-by-word reader to immediately begin to read fluidly. In fact, I've seen many children who can suddenly read two or three grade levels higher as soon as they put those lenses on! (Check Appendix B for an optometrist in your area who will prescribe Plus Lenses.)

Tips to Reduce the Stress of Reading

It's a good idea to remove your corrective lenses while reading, especially if you're nearsighted. The ideal position at which to hold a book is the distance that creates the least physiological stress. This is usually the distance between the bottom knuckle of your middle finger and your elbow. If you can't see clearly at that distance without your glasses, place your book where you can read it easily and move it a little closer to the ideal position each day.

Your book should also be at a slant parallel to the plane of your face. A tilt-top book holder or desk is helpful to keep the book at the correct angle. It's easy to make your own reading stand. You will need two standard-size doorstops and a 12″ by 18″ firm wooden board with a smooth surface. Attach (screw in) the doorstops to the board at a right angle, as shown in the illustration below. To use, simply set the board down on a table or desk so that it slopes down toward you (the two doorstops will be on the side farthest away from you). Then place your reading material on the board.

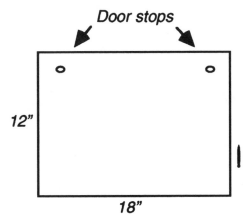

The Reading Table

Use a "Look Up" Bookmark

This wonderful tool prevents overconcentration during reading or studying, by keeping the eyes relaxed and the field open. I wish it could be taught to all children as soon as they enter elementary school. I believe that if it were, it would go a long way to reducing the incidence of myopia in school-age children. It's a fun way to get all the readers in your family into the habit of looking up periodically:

Using a piece of thin cardboard, make everyone in the family a personalized bookmark that says, "Stop. Look up. Look away. Breathe! Now put me two pages ahead." Place this bookmark in the book two pages ahead of the page you are on, and follow the instructions every time you reach it.

Another tip that will encourage you to look up while reading is to place your desk or reading chair so that it faces into a room or out of a window—not against a wall. The farther you can see, the better. While reading or doing paperwork, occasionally look up at a distant

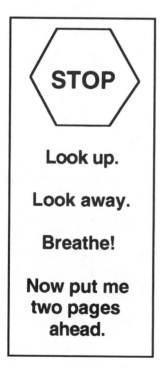

"Look Up!" Bookmark

object and allow it to come into clear focus, then switch into Open Focus for a moment.

How to Avoid "Terminal" Illness

Working at a computer screen is rapidly becoming a major contributor to visual stress in the emerging communications age. If you regularly work or play in front of a computer terminal, you are already aware how quickly your eyes become fatigued and strained. Have you also noticed that when you get up from the screen, you can't see as clearly as you could before?

Although a wide range of health hazards have begun to be associated with visual display terminals, the visual aspect of what I call "terminal" illness is simply a new version of near-point stress. Our eyes operate most effortlessly when their lines of sight are parallel or slightly diverged, as they do naturally when we are viewing a distant scene. As soon as we try to focus on anything much closer than twenty feet, our eyes must begin to converge, which takes effort to maintain.

At the distance of the typical computer screen, the resulting convergence (and effort) is quite strong. When this short-range focus is maintained for hours without a break, it creates stress throughout the mind/body—our muscles tighten, our breath becomes shallow, our attention wanders, our vision weakens . . . we feel mentally, emotionally, and physically drained. The more time we spend at the computer, the more this short-range view tends to become imprinted in our system, making it difficult to reexpand our focus to resume distance vision—and as our lines of sight fall inward, so does our entire being.

This constriction is further aggravated by the unnaturally fast pace and high stress of many video display terminal jobs. Yet even those who must use a computer all day long can begin to counteract its effects with a few basic steps:

1. Don't strain to see. The artificial light of a video screen may still be hard to see even after you no longer need your glasses for other near-point activities. Don't hesitate to use

the *minimum* prescription you need to avoid squinting and straining while you work. Remind yourself to breathe fully and blink frequently to avoid staring.

2. Use the passive seeing meditation (page 106) to keep your eyes flexible and active. Whenever possible, take a visual break: Shift your eyes from side to side, top to bottom, and corner to corner of the screen. Then alternate looking at the screen and away from it, ideally into the distance (as described above for reading) several times.

3. Make yourself a reminder card that says, "Stop. Look up. Look away. Breathe!" and post it on or near your screen, where you will see it frequently. This will remind you to breathe with awareness and to look up whenever you can. Throughout the day, *take advantage of every opportunity to use your long-distance vision.*

4. Give your vision frequent mini-vacations: Shift into Open Focus by expanding your awareness to your entire visual field. This is helpful even if you can only do it for a few moments while you continue to work. Every time that you have an extra minute or so, give yourself a palming break (page 103).

5. Improve the ambient light: If possible, change the lighting around your work area to natural sunlight or "full-spectrum" lights that simulate natural sunlight. For instance, if you work at home, see if it's possible to move your computer to a window. Even in a large windowless office, you may be able to place a small full-spectrum lamp at your workstation. During breaks or lunch, try to find some direct sunlight (not through a window) and practice the palming and sunning meditations (pages 103 and 104).

Try Pinhole Glasses

Pinhole glasses, based on a discovery by Leonardo da Vinci, are a fun vision-support tool for many kinds of focusing problems. They consist of eyeglass frames fitted with black plastic lenses pierced by many small holes that focus light onto the retina. Pinholes allow

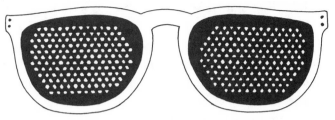

Pinhole Glasses

the habitual lens wearer to experience significantly clearer vision—without wearing prescription lenses (see Appendix A for more information).

Pinholes work by only allowing parallel light rays to enter the eyes, so that less focusing is necessary. The experience of improved vision without prescriptions, straining, or staring can feel like a major breakthrough.

When you first put them on, pinholes can feel like magic—"I can see clearly without my correction!" They also look intriguing, and can be fun to wear. However, since the black screen restricts your visual field, they should not be used all day long, at night, or while driving. It's also important to remember that pinholes themselves don't create a permanent improvement in your unaided vision. They can, however, be a great transitional tool to help you reduce the amount of time that you wear prescription lenses. For instance, some people like to use them to watch television or movies without corrective lenses while they are recovering their clear eyesight.

Remove Your Sunglasses

Sunglasses, first developed for airplane pilots during World War I, were popularized by Hollywood war movies. I've found that the regular use of sunglasses desensitizes the photoreceptors in the eyes, thereby creating a hypersensitivity to light. Paradoxically, sunglasses also suppress the signals that let you know when the light actually *is* too bright to tolerate—the rare occasions when you might *really* need sunglasses, such as on the beach or when skiing down a snow-covered mountain on a really bright day.

If you habitually wear sunglasses, your eyes' ability to recognize and adjust to variations in light has been greatly reduced. However, they will begin to regain their normal adaptability as soon as you start weaning yourself from overuse of sunglasses. When you do need to wear sunglasses, switch to a neutral gray tint. Trendy colors, such as yellow, pink, blue, and red, are especially hard on the eyes and may have other detrimental health effects.

I've also recently begun to see small children and even infants wearing sunglasses, apparently as a result of media reports on the growing dangers of UV light. I would strongly advise against putting sunglasses on any child, except under very unusual circumstances. The long-term effects that wearing sunglasses might have on a child's development are simply not yet understood, and research has shown that our eyes must absorb the full spectrum of natural light (including UV) for optimal physical health. (My first book, *Light: Medicine of the Future*, has much more information on this research and on the effects of wearing sunglasses.)

The habit of wearing tinted glasses or sunglasses indoors as well as outdoors is especially detrimental, as it not only dramatically reduces the amount of light that the eyes receive but also distorts the natural spectral balance contained in sunlight. That's why I don't recommend the use of photochromic lenses, which automatically darken whenever you encounter brighter light. Adaptation to light is a natural, intended function of the eyes. Why substitute a pair of artificial lenses for a task that the eyes are already exquisitely designed to perform?

So to improve your vision, remove your tinted lenses and sunglasses (just as you remove your corrective lenses). When you first remove them, your eyes will probably feel especially sensitive to light. Regular practice of the sunning meditation (page 104) can rapidly strengthen your light tolerance during that transition. There is nothing wrong with occasionally wearing sunglasses on an especially bright day—just don't do it every time you go out in the sun. The less you wear sunglasses, the less you will need them—and the more light your eyes will be able to tolerate without straining.

9 A Day in the Life of Your New Vision

Even if you're on the right track,
you'll get run over if you just sit there.
—Will Rogers

FOR MANY PEOPLE, the biggest hurdle to trying something new is just starting it. So I'd like to take you step by step through a hypothetical day without your glasses. When you take off your glasses, your entire routine may feel new. You may even feel that you are having to relearn the simplest activities. Instead of considering this to be a handicap—for example, "I'm absolutely *blind* without my glasses!"—realize that it offers you the opportunity to develop a meditative, conscious awareness in all your activities.

I suggest that you first choose a day during which you can follow your own timing and be fully aware of each moment without having to rush—such as a weekend day. Consider this a sacred time to be with yourself. The more aware you can be, the more you will get out of this process. If you are thinking about the past or the future, you won't really be seeing and feeling what is happening now. Once you have practiced removing your glasses on the weekend a few times, try integrating it into your usual workday. The example below includes situations that you may encounter on both a weekend and a weekday.

Let's start at the beginning of the day. Every morning when we awaken we have an opportunity to consciously restore our vision, our relationship to life: How do you feel as you open your eyes? Do you feel peaceful or urgent, as if life is rushing by you? Become aware of your breathing. Allow yourself to let go of any intentions to do or accomplish anything.

As you lie in bed, gaze softly up toward the ceiling. Shift into Open Focus, and allow your eyes to move freely. Simply notice whatever you are seeing, whether it is clear or blurry. If there are any noises or distractions, just let them flow by you. Notice how different this feels from your normal awareness. Can you sense the openness of your energy field?

Continue to gaze toward the ceiling, allowing your eyes to flow into an endless dance. Remember the breath awareness and palming meditations (page 97 and 103)? You'll be using them throughout the day. You can start right now. You can also practice seeing the flash (page 91) as well as any other eye meditations you enjoy.

When you feel ready, gently get out of bed, maintaining that soft awareness. Don't put on your glasses or contacts. Walk gently to the bathroom, continuing to notice how peaceful you feel. Notice that you are seeing exactly what you need to see. Perform your usual morning activities while breathing effortlessly. Allow yourself to move at a slow, comfortable pace.

Then begin to get dressed. Notice what you choose to wear. Is it difficult to select your outfit without lenses? Are you drawn toward different clothes than you typically choose? Are you wondering whether your clothes will look wrinkled or won't match? Are you wondering whether you will be able to present yourself to the world without your lenses? Notice everything you are feeling while you stay with your breath.

After getting dressed, take that soft awareness outside and connect with Nature. Feel the earth beneath your feet and the breeze as it touches your body. Breathe in the fresh air and Nature's sounds and smells. Notice the sky and the sun overhead. Greet the sun with any ritual you like and do your sunning exercise. If you're in a big city, do you have a balcony or an open window through which you can welcome the sun? Is there a park nearby? No matter where you live, there are generally more opportunities for contact with Nature than you may think there are.

Now look around you. At first you may only notice that your new vision is blurry, and you may miss some of the things you're used to seeing. Rather than noticing what you *can't* see, notice what you *can* see. Some people find that color and depth perception are much better without their glasses.

Take a short walk, maintaining an open awareness. Breathe and do Open Focus, so that the walk becomes a moving meditation. Allow your eyes to see for you, without judging your sight as clear or blurry. See the following chapter, "How to Take a Vision Walk," for more suggestions.

By now you may be starting to think about eating. Tune in and discover if you're really hungry or if you're simply seeking food to alleviate feelings of anxiety. If you're not really hungry yet, you might want to write about your feelings and experiences (see page 146 for more about keeping a journal) or extend your walk in the fresh air. Whatever you do, stay with your breath and your feelings. Don't blur them out.

How long has it been since you had a meal without your corrective lenses? If you're a hard-core lens-wearer, it may have been several years. However, you won't eat the wrong foods if you're not wearing your glasses, just as you didn't dress in the wrong clothes. Continue to breathe gently and do Open Focus as you choose, prepare, and eat your meal. Notice how different the kitchen feels without your glasses. It may take a little more time to prepare the food, so go easy with yourself.

When you're ready to eat, sit in a quiet spot and place your full attention on eating, using all your senses. Don't read the paper, watch TV, or engage in an animated conversation while eating. These habits reduce awareness and may contribute to poor digestion. Notice how you're eating. Are you eating more slowly than usual? Does the food taste any different? How does your stomach feel as you eat? Mindful eating is a mini-meditation that is especially helpful for people who have weight problems, digestive difficulties, or eating disorders.

Eating is another aspect of life that we may blur out as we focus on more "important" things. Yet how can the nourishment of our tissues be unimportant? You may have heard the saying "You are what you eat." Sometimes I wonder if it's more accurate to say "You are *how* you eat." How often do we eat with gratitude and awareness of the gift of food? How often do we rush through the meal as if it's an unpleasant chore, while distracting ourselves as much as possible? I wonder if this lack of awareness could be a major factor in the current epidemic of imbalances related to digestion, weight, and eating habits.

Now it's time to see how it feels to go into the world without your glasses. You may be driving to work, visiting friends, running errands, or just experimenting. If you're walking or taking public transportation, carry your glasses on a chain or someplace where you can easily reach them. Put them on only when you really need to—to make sure you're getting on the right bus or subway, for example. Otherwise, continue to notice how different the world looks through your natural sight. Whenever you begin to feel anxious, *breathe* and shift into Open Focus instead of automatically reaching for those lenses.

If you'll be driving, go and sit in the car. Take off your glasses and place them on the seat beside you. For many people, discovering that they can drive without corrective lenses is the most profound shift in the entire vision improvement process. Sooner or later, you may feel confident enough in your improving eyesight to take this step. But right now, just take a few moments and visualize a new way of driving:

Begin by remembering the last few times you drove while wearing your lenses. You could see very clearly, but how did you feel? Were you stressed and hurried? Were your shoulders tense? Did you clutch the steering wheel tightly? Were you driving faster than you should have been? Were you really attending to the road, or was your mind racing ahead? If you were thinking about what was going to happen when you reached your destination, or what had happened before you left, then your eyes were darting all over your visual field, looking up memories and creating new images. Your eyes were too busy to scan the road. Your attention was somewhere else. I've found that most auto accidents occur because we're *not present*, not because we can't see. Even after a near miss, we may find ourselves wondering, "How did that happen? What *was* I thinking of?"

Now, still sitting in the car, *visualize* yourself driving down the road without your lenses, seeing clearly and feeling relaxed and effortless. See yourself breathing and driving mindfully as you easily hold the steering wheel, press the gas pedal, and allow your eyes to scan the road. Let your awareness slow down to the moment. Allow yourself to be totally aware. Enjoy driving at a speed that feels safe and comfortable.

How different does this feel from your last visualization? Which one feels safer?

You haven't put your glasses on yet. Look around and assess the situation. How well are you seeing right now? Do you need your glasses to drive out of the garage or driveway? Are you driving right into heavy traffic, or are you on a quiet country lane? Notice the part of you that feels anxious and spend a few minutes breathing with that fear.

Of course, before driving without your glasses, make sure you can drive safely. Consult your natural vision improvement practitioner for a prescription strength that best supports your vision while keeping you within the legal requirements for driving. You may then decide to wear a reduced prescription or even go without your glasses—but be sure to drive responsibly! You don't need to prove anything to yourself by driving without glasses. If you have any doubt at all, leave your lenses on while driving until you feel confident that you can see clearly enough to drive safely while wearing a reduced prescription.

If you're not ready to drive with a weaker correction, you can pretend that you're learning to drive—with your glasses on, take the car out on a Sunday and find an empty parking lot. Remove your glasses when you get there and practice driving around the lot while you breathe, blink, and do Open Focus. Then put them back on when you're ready to drive home. Remember, there's no reason to rush yourself into driving without them.

When you do begin to drive without your glasses, keep breathing and put them back on whenever you need to. Notice whenever you begin to feel anxious. What is that discomfort about? How much of it is that you really can't see well, and how much of it is fearful anticipation or conditioning? You can put your glasses back on at any time; just do it with *awareness* rather than denial of your feelings.

If you've been driving with your lenses on, take them off again *as soon as you park the car.* How does your vision look now compared to how it looked when you woke up this morning? Notice how much blurrier things are after you've worn your glasses for even a few minutes. As you take your glasses on and off throughout the day, keep noticing how your vision shifts.

As you walk down the street, remember to breathe mindfully and practice Open Focus. Notice how different everyone looks, and how they seem to be looking at you differently, too. It isn't because you look better without your glasses. When you surrender your corrective lenses, your field expands and you enter a state of relaxed openness, which is very attractive to others. Deep inside we would all like to be that open.

Now let's imagine that you're going to work today. Most people will be able to practice breath awareness, Open Focus, palming, and tracing while working, or at least during breaks in their day. You can practice these "vision meditations" when you go to the bathroom, before and after lunch, between clients or classes, and so on. If your day consists mostly of near-point work—reading, doing paperwork, working at a computer—it's important to remind yourself to look up periodically. You can put a little sign on your desk or computer that says, "Look up. Look away. Breathe!" If your day consists mostly of working with other people, continually remind yourself to breathe and trace the faces you are looking at.

Rather than feeling uncomfortable because your coworkers might wonder what you're doing, share your experiment with them. Some may not understand what you're doing, but very likely others will be curious and want to try it, too. You can tell them about your experiences and encourage their interest. Such support will help you all to progress faster.

Sooner or later during the day, you may suddenly find yourself face-to-face with all your anxieties and doubts. It can feel as if you're "hitting the wall"—like an addict experiencing an urgent need for his next cigarette, drink, or drug . . . except that you'll be reaching for your prescription lenses instead of a chemical.

By this time you are probably well past the point when you would have normally put on your glasses. Before you react, allow yourself to fully *feel* your feelings. Do you feel vulnerable, helpless, impatient, angry? Whatever it is, know that you don't have to push that feeling away anymore. Notice and breathe with it, *allowing yourself to feel whatever you're feeling.*

By now your mind has probably thought of a dozen reasons why you should simply put your glasses back on and forget this whole thing: "What's so bad about wearing glasses? This is just too uncomfortable, and anyway, I'll never be able to shift my vision. I'll just resign myself to wearing glasses for the rest of my life." Notice those thoughts and remember that you don't have to believe them, change them, argue with them, or do anything about them. Simply acknowledge them and allow them to pass spontaneously. Also, writing in a journal can be a very helpful exercise to release those emotional pressures (see page 146).

By taking off your glasses, you automatically access a greater sensitivity, a greater openness. At first, it may feel like fear, discomfort, or vulnerability—but it is also gentleness, laughter, joy, relaxation. Most people feel softer, less intense, more easygoing without their glasses. At some point, ask your family, friends, or coworkers to compare what you are like with your glasses on and with them off.

The next time you're having a heartfelt conversation or trying to share a deep feeling, take your glasses off and notice what happens. Most people say they can experience and express their emotions far more easily with their glasses off! Once you've felt the difference, you'll automatically remove your glasses whenever you want to communicate from the heart.

If you're a therapist or a healer, or if your work involves personal communication, you'll find it helpful to remove your glasses as much as possible while you work. You may *think* you'll see less that way, but if you experiment, you may actually notice that you can listen better, communicate better, feel more, and simply be far more present without your glasses.

If your work involves driving or other hazardous activities, you may need to reduce your prescription very gradually to maintain a safe working environment. Abide by any regulations that require you to wear corrective lenses. Just make sure that you aren't over-correcting your vision—wear the minimum prescription that you need for safety and legality, not the maximum! Even if you must wear your glasses at work, take advantage of every opportunity to take them off: breaks, weekends, after work, vacations. Remember that your willingness to change and awareness that you *can* change are the most important elements of vision improvement.

As the day goes on and we get physically tired, our vision also gets tired—so be patient with yourself toward the end of the day. As the sunlight dims, many people find that they need to give their eyesight more support. Even if you drove to work in the morning with a reduced prescription, you may need to wear a stronger one to drive home at night. When you get home, remove your glasses right away and take another walk. Keep breathing, blinking, and practicing Open Focus. Before you come inside, do your evening sunning exercise.

If you're driving or walking after dark, notice how different your vision feels at night. Many of us were afraid of the dark as children, and people who live in cities sometimes just don't feel safe going out on a dark street. We don't usually think about how those fears may be affecting our vision. The combination of fear of the dark and the fact that our peripheral vision is dominant at night means that we are much more in touch with our feelings at night than in the daytime. If we aren't comfortable having those feelings, our night vision will probably be weak.

To improve your night vision, practice walking and looking around in the dark. You don't have to walk very far, but do walk in a place that feels safe. At night, we primarily see with our peripheral vision, not our central focus, so practice Open Focus to see in the dark, rather than trying to "zoom in" on objects as in the daytime.

If you like, practice some of the vision meditations in the evening. Do Open Focus and palming as your last activities before going to bed, just as they were your first activities in the morning. Then fall effortlessly into a restful, deep sleep, and in your dreams, sooner or later, you'll find yourself seeing with a clarity beyond anything you've ever dreamed before.

10 How to Take a Vision Walk

Life is a journey, not a destination.
—Dr. Robert Anthony

WE'VE BEEN looking at the profound connection between vision and awareness, but vision is *movement,* as well. How our eyes see is reflected in how our body moves, and vice versa. Vision is actually more of an active sense than a receptive one. We assume that we simply receive visual information through our eyes, but seeing is actually far more complex than that. What we see is the interpretation that our brain has made from light impulses sent from our eyes. The brain doesn't hesitate to improvise and "fill in" any apparently missing information.

Furthermore, the eyes are our navigational system. They are the aspect of the brain that we use to orient ourselves in the world. Every physical move is directed by our visual orientation to the world. The next time you observe an athlete, notice how her every move is guided by her visual awareness. Even supposedly "blind" people have to visualize themselves in relation to the physical world in order to get around. When we evaluate vision without movement, we are observing only a fraction of our visual sense. Our visual relationship to the world shapes our physical posture, from head to toe.

That's why taking a daily walk is one of the most powerful "eye meditations" you can do. Walking also brings us into appreciation of the life force that surrounds us, and allows us to merge our field with a greater whole. As our eyes are filled with the beauty and energy around us, they are motivated to open up and see even more.

Although walking is an excellent form of exercise that benefits all aspects of the body/mind, here we will be focusing on how to use it as a meditation for shifting our inner and outer vision. If you are already walking regularly, try a few of these suggestions on your next outing. If you aren't in the habit of walking, it can be fun to get together with a friend who also wears glasses to try these "eye meditations" together. You can even form a support group of people who meet to take a vision walk together every morning or evening.

Selecting Your Path

Choosing the place where you will walk is as important as choosing the place where you would do any other meditation. You will want to walk in a relatively undisturbed setting—a quiet country lane is ideal! If that is not readily available, try to get out of town as often as you can on weekends and holidays. If you live in a city, a large park or a quiet residential street may be good places to walk.

I live in the Colorado Rockies, where we are always walking either downhill or uphill. You'll find you get the greatest benefit from walking paths that contain upgrades and downgrades, not because of the cardiovascular workout but because this "awareness exercise" involves your attitudes about walking up and down. The experience of walking uphill and downhill adds a key psychological component to the walk, a powerful point of access to your fears and self-limitations. You can gradually build up to steeper inclines if you aren't used to them. But unless you have a potentially dangerous health condition, I would encourage you to start walking along a hilly path anyway, and just go at your own pace (as with any exercise program, consult your doctor before beginning if there is any doubt about your physical fitness). If there are no hills around your home, try to find a steeper place to walk on weekends.

It's also important to walk in an area with open views, so that you can feel the full expanse of your visual and energetic field. If you are myopic, this is especially important. Nearsighted people often limit themselves to near-point visual activities and avoid open areas, which may be subtly threatening to them. Most people who live indoor lifestyles in crowded cities and suburbs rarely see the full expanse of the earth from horizon to horizon—except maybe on television or in the movies. A person living in the middle of a large city can only see far away by looking straight up at a narrow piece of sky, or by going to the top of a skyscraper—but you can't take a walk up there!

You won't be wearing any corrective lenses during your vision walk, but if it feels too scary to leave them at home, just put your glasses in your pocket or on a chain around your neck. Then, any time you feel the urge to put them on during the walk, ask yourself whether you really need them or whether you're simply feeling some anxiety.

If you normally wear sunglasses while walking, try leaving them off during your vision walk. The more you leave your sunglasses off, the faster your eyes will regain their natural light tolerance. Instead, wear a hat or a visor, and eventually you will want to leave these light shields at home, too, except on very sunny days. You can become just as addicted to them as you can to sunglasses or corrective lenses. To restimulate your eyes' natural tolerance of sunlight, practice sunning and palming (see pages 104 and 103) before, during, and after walking.

Walking Meditation

This walk is a kind of moving meditation. Begin to move easily and rhythmically. Turn your attention to your breath and allow your awareness to gently move into Open Focus. Whenever you notice yourself thinking, allow that mental chatter to be a signal to gently return your attention to your breath. The more we think, the harder it is to breathe, but breathing becomes lighter and easier as we return to Open Focus and breath awareness.

Thoughts are like clouds moving through the sky of our awareness. Sometimes we confuse the clouds with the sky—we think that our thoughts *are* our awareness. In Open Focus, all your thoughts can pass effortlessly through you.

While walking in Open Focus, allow your eyes to trace everything you see (page 99). It doesn't matter if you can see clearly, just visually outline everything within view. Notice that as you trace a mysterious blur you may suddenly get a clear flash or an intuitive sense of what it might be. Keep your eyes moving continuously. Notice how much you are able to see rather than how much you can't see. Also notice whether you are perceiving anything in the "invisible" air.

The natural rhythm of walking feet is a beautiful movement that we usually either take for granted or hurry along. Take a moment now to fully appreciate it. Allow your feet to move easily and gracefully: As the foot leaves the ground, the ankle disengages. Instead of rushing to put the foot back down, allow the ankle to release smoothly. As the foot approaches the ground, it "looks down," as if there were eyes on the bottom of the foot (only the eyes on the foot look down, not the eyes in the head). Then allow your heel to gently "touch down," followed by the rest of your foot.

Notice how your entire body wants to move rhythmically and gracefully. Just as you allow your eyes to see for you, allow your feet to walk for you and your arms to flow at your sides. Look at nothing as your eyes keep dancing around. Breathe gently and notice any feelings or sensations that come up.

Where Are You Headed?

As you walk, bring your attention to the upper part of your body—your head and neck. Imagine that your head is balanced on a movable pivot at the top of your spine. As you move, allow your head and neck to gently bobble on that point. Now visualize that your head is slowly floating higher. Your body is still grounded, but your neck is getting longer and longer. Your head is moving up to about five feet above your body. Walk for a while with a five-foot neck topped by a gently balanced head. What does that feel like?

Then allow your neck to slowly telescope even farther, until your head is ten feet above your body. The rest of your body remains in relaxed and effortless motion. Sense as tangibly as possible what your head feels like floating ten feet up in the air. When I do this I feel very free, very open, far removed from my usual mental pressures.

Now notice the position of your head and eyes. As the leading edge of our navigational system, the eyes show us where we are "headed." This inner orientation begins in our feelings and attitudes and manifests as our posture and the direction of our gaze. You can easily observe how people often walk looking downward, with their head slightly forward. When the head is down, it restricts the breath at the throat. Have you ever noticed that it is harder to speak while looking down? As soon as your head goes back up, your throat and your breath open up. You begin moving forward again, breathing easier and taking in more of life. So it's important to allow your feet to see for you as you walk. Don't look down; let your feet discover how to find their own way!

This is not just a physical change. As the body shifts, how we see ourselves in relation to the world changes. Walking in a new position may bring up feelings—fear, anger, or insecurity—that have been "hiding" inside the old posture. Just notice how it feels to walk with your head up and how it feels when you move your head back to its familiar position. Is there a difference? Does the discomfort or fear seem to go away when your head is up?

As you walk, keep your plane of view parallel to the ground—don't look down in front of you to check the path! Raise your eyes and look straight ahead. If the path is *really* rough or rocky, keep your focus about ten feet in front of you, not at your feet. Continue to relax, breathe, and practice Open Focus, and you'll see all that you need to see. Notice that now you feel taller, can see more, and that your lungs have expanded. Notice how your view of life changes when you shift the direction of your gaze. If you tend to feel small, helpless, and frightened, notice how moving your eyes up reframes that contracted point of view.

The Eyes in the Back of Your Head

Now turn around and walk backward, facing the way you have come (skip this if it is too uncomfortable). Imagine that you have eyes in the back of your head, which are looking in the opposite direction from your physical eyes. Allow the eyes in the back of your head to guide your feet forward. Notice any changes in your posture or your feelings.

Try this while you are walking uphill and notice the difference between walking uphill forward and walking uphill backward. People usually say that when they walk uphill backward they don't get as winded and their heart doesn't beat as fast. Their muscles seem to work more effortlessly, as if nothing is interfering with them.

We seem to believe that walking uphill is hard, that it is a struggle. As long as our physical eyes can see that we are headed uphill, the body responds accordingly. However, as soon as we turn around, even though we are still walking uphill, our eyes are looking downhill. We believe that walking downhill is easy! So it feels like a completely different experience. Our sense of uphill struggle is no longer activated. It's also true that when we turn around we begin using a different set of muscles, but even so we can see how much of the difficulty of walking uphill is created by our own beliefs.

After walking backward, turn sideways so that your whole body is facing right. Now begin to walk up the hill crabwise while still facing sideways—crossing your right foot in front of your left, and then your left foot behind your right as you walk up the hill. When that feels comfortable, turn around and do it while facing the other side. Continue to stay in Open Focus and breathe mindfully. This is a practice of physical coordination in a meditative state.

Spinning

Now you can do some paradoxical movement exercises. These visualizations disengage the linear mind because it can't keep track of what is going on. You will keep walking forward (or backward), while visualizing your body spinning or rotating. This really gets you into Open Focus and conscious breathing! The nonlinear activity removes your attention from the chronic tension of trying to see, at which point you may really begin to see for the first time. Don't take this too seriously, don't turn it into a task—just have fun with it!

First, while walking forward or backward, begin to visualize that your body is spinning slowly to the right. The idea is to actually feel your body gently turning. See yourself turning around as vividly as you can as you continue to walk. After you have been spinning to the right for a few moments, reverse the motion—imagine yourself turning to the left for a while.

Now walk forward and imagine that you are doing back flips—see your body actually flipping over backward as you walk. This is a very interesting sensation. Your mind/body may initially be confused by the instructions to move forward while simultaneously spinning backward. Then walk backward and see your body flipping over forward. Notice whether your body responds or your posture changes.

Now, while walking, visualize your head slowly spinning all around to the right while your body continues to move forward. This is like unscrewing your head from your body. How does that feel, especially around your throat? Next, do it counterclockwise: Move forward and visualize your head slowly turning 360 degrees around to the left.

Once you get the idea, you can make up all kinds of other paradoxical visualizations. Just remember to keep having fun!

The last practice is very important: Start skipping! As you skip, begin to laugh as hard as you can. If you are walking with friends, join hands while skipping and laughing out loud. Do that for a while. Skipping and laughing and doing Open Focus.

This walk will not be boring!

A vision walk really *can* improve your vision, especially when you do it regularly. Even one vision walk can produce a measurable shift in your eyesight. In 1991, I visited Dr. Wanda Tort in Puerto Rico. Wanda is an optometrist who had been trying to reduce her prescription for some time. I suggested that we go for a vision walk. She recalls what happened:

> During the walk I took off my glasses and we did Open Focus and other strange things. We were walking backwards and visualizing that we were spinning and looking through the back of our heads.

Then Jacob suddenly asked me if I could see the numbers on a license plate some distance away. I said, "No!" I thought, That's impossible! I said what I thought it was, anyway—this all happened so fast that I didn't have time to think about it. Then we walked up to the car, pacing off the distance. It was about ninety feet, and I had got it absolutely right. I couldn't believe it. I just couldn't believe that I had read it correctly from that far away. I thought it was my imagination, or just a lucky guess.

We went back to the office. Jacob examined me, and found that I was able to see 20/20 with one third the prescription that I had been wearing. That was hard to believe, but most of the time now I wear lenses that are half as strong as I was wearing then, and I can see a perfect 20/20 with them.

Walking and practicing the eye meditations show our eyes how to see more effortlessly. How can we begin to see, think, and live effortlessly all the time? How can we start trusting our innate genius? I've found that one of the most important elements is *Open Living*—being present and staying current in everything we do.

11 Living Clearly: Being Present and Staying Current

We are healed of a suffering only by experiencing it to the full.
— *Marcel Proust*

REMOVING OUR corrective lenses reveals the difficult feelings we were trying to avoid when we first got them. Usually, these are childhood feelings that we have more or less avoided our entire adult life, even if we've had years of therapy. As long as we're wearing glasses or contacts, we're carrying around an invisible barrier to recognizing and resolving some of our deepest issues. Those lenses tend to hold our awareness in the shape of our unresolved fear or anxiety. One of my patients who was reducing her prescription noticed that

> my prescription was like a snapshot of who I thought I was and what I thought the world was—my relationship to others—at any given moment. As my prescription increased, it seemed to be measuring a contraction or closing down of who I thought I was. When I started reducing my prescription by using glasses of different strengths, I noticed that whenever I would wear an old, stronger pair again, I would return to the more contracted mind-set that it had locked me into.

It is very difficult to really expand one's vision while continuing to see the world through a pair of blinders. To evolve and heal, we must begin to see as freely and innocently as a child. A participant in one of my workshops commented that about 80 percent of the people [in the group] had some vision improvement—quite a bit of improvement, most of them. Emotional awareness seemed to be what was creating the changes. That inspired me to look at the emotional aspect of my own vision. I think that emotional release is 100 percent of the change. I guess all I am doing is becoming more aware of my emotions—what I am feeling and why I am not living life.

One thing that really sticks in my mind is that quote [from the Talmud], "We do not see things as they are. We see them as we are." If we don't see clearly, it is because we are not clear.

When we remove our lenses, our hidden emotions reappear and we need to find a new way of relating to them without "blurring out." It can be fascinating and empowering to become reacquainted with the aspect of yourself that has been hiding behind your glasses. However, that part of you may also be hard to identify at first, since it has been invisible for so long.

Writing Your Vision History

You may want to begin keeping a "vision journal," and record there all the impressions, memories, feelings, and dreams that are triggered as you remove your corrective lenses. You can begin the journal with your "vision history."

Your vision history is an account of everything that you feel, remember, or know about your relationship to your vision up to now. It can start with your earliest visual memories, and move on to describe the events that occurred around or just before the time you got your first pair of glasses. What feelings did you have about those events? How did you react to those feelings? (If you can't remember much, the next visualization, "Seeing the Hidden You," can help start the flow of memories.)

Can you remember each time your prescription changed? What was happening in your life each time your vision seemed to get worse? If you're an adult, you've probably had more eye exams than you can count. What have your experiences and feelings been about eye doctors and eye exams? How do you feel about wearing glasses in general? Has it changed over the years? How long do you wear your lenses each day? Do you wear them for all activities or selectively? How do you feel about your vision in general? Is it a source of pride, shame, or any other strong feeling?

Seeing the Hidden You

Your vision is constantly in flux, continually evolving, but your corrective lenses are fixed. They are still casting your vision of reality into the shape of the events you "couldn't face" when you first got them. Here's a visualization to help you reconnect with the "hidden you":

Take off your glasses or contacts and close your eyes. Bring your attention to your breath. Breathe freely, with awareness of any tension, until you feel ready for the next step.

Now think of a time in your childhood when you were really happy. When was that? How old were you? When you find it, feel and reexperience it.

What was happening in your life then? What were you feeling? What were you happy about? Try to recall as much as you can about that time.

Visualize your face at that time. Are you smiling? Look into your eyes. Are they happy? Is there a sparkle, a glimmer of joy in them? Take a moment to enjoy that memory

Now bring your attention back to your breath for a few moments. When you feel centered, think back to when you first noticed a difference in your vision, or when you received your first glasses. When was that? How old were you? When you find it, feel and re-experience it.

What was happening in your life then? What were you feeling? What were you angry, sad, or happy about? Try to recall as much as you can about that time. If you have difficulty remembering, just allow your mind to be present with it. A memory will probably come up if you give it a chance.

Visualize your face at that time. Are you smiling? Look into your eyes. Is there still a sparkle, a glimmer of joy in them? Are they happy? What is the difference in your eyes and in your life between the two scenes?

Can you remember the emotional issues that were going on then?

Do you feel that you were able to resolve them? Do you feel that those issues are still affecting your life?

Every person I have worked with has been able to uncover some kind of major emotional stress in the one- to two-year period before their vision first deteriorated. This visualization can give you a sense of the stress that was too difficult to face, the feelings that your glasses have helped you to suppress. As you begin to remove your glasses, those feelings will come up again, either from within or (apparently) through external events. When they do, your initial response will probably be an urge to put your glasses back on (or wear stronger glasses)—but that will simply reinforce your old way of being.

When you did the visualization, did you find that your memories of that time were blurry or unclear? Or were they so painful that you really didn't want to (or couldn't) remember them? Have you literally "blurred out" that period of your life? If you answer "yes" to any of these questions, it indicates that the emotional issues of that time are still unresolved. If you're willing to take the time to reopen those memories and associations, you'll begin to *see* and *heal* the part of your life experience that you've hidden for so long.

You can use this visualization as a starting point to reflect further on what was going on then. Were you happy at home? Did you feel loved? Did you feel safe? Who was your biggest enemy? Had you recently experienced . . .

- the death of a friend or family member?
- a move or change of school or friends?
- a divorce?
- a new sibling or change in family members?
- shame or embarrassment?
- emotional or physical abuse?

You may know that one or more of these events occurred around that time, and still be unable to remember how they affected you. However, any of these events would be a major stressor for a child.

The inability to remember childhood stress may be a way to protect yourself from feeling the fear or pain that was associated with it. If you find it hard to remember the events, tune into any feelings that come up about that time, and trust that they have some meaning for your vision. It's not really necessary to know exactly what happened as long as you can tune into the emotional tone of that time.

Expressing Your Feelings

Whether or not you can remember the specific events, your eyesight and your lenses are still a perfect mold of your defensive posture back then, even if your prescription has changed considerably in the intervening years. Once you have an idea of what those feelings were, consider how they are affecting your life now. Do you still feel unloved, unsafe, abandoned, abused, ashamed? How are you dealing with those feelings now? Do you tend to block them out or project them onto other people? Do you simply ignore them and hope they'll go away?

To get and keep a significant vision improvement, you need to develop a new way of relating to those feelings. The most powerful step you can take is very simple: communication. Communication doesn't just mean going to see a therapist once a week (although that can be very helpful). The idea is to train yourself away from the habit of hiding your feelings inside or pushing them out onto others. Communication really means learning a new way to relate to life.

The habit of sharing your feelings when they are fresh, no matter how angry, shameful, or painful they are, is probably the most important thing you can do to clear your internal and external blur. If you're not feeling okay about an experience, express it! Share your feelings with the people who are directly involved, not just your best friend or your therapist. It's not helpful to accuse or blame someone else because *you* feel upset. Share your experience and then listen without judgment while the other person responds. Communication is not about figuring out who is right and who is wrong—everyone sees the world differently, and both of you are right to feel whatever you are feeling.

It seems that the natural impulse of all emotions is to simply move through us. It's only when we hold them within that they get stuck. A strong feeling can be left unexpressed only if an effort is made to suppress its spontaneous manifestation. That effort narrows our energetic field and diminishes our vision. To release those suppressed feelings, we must learn to express our pain, anger, and fear.

Every time we express ourselves, we lose a little more emotional clutter. It's like taking out the garbage. If your back porch is full of trash, it may take you a while to clear it out, but once you've cleaned it up, you only have to deal with one piece of litter at a time. You never have to clean off the entire porch again, because you are no longer allowing the garbage to accumulate.

The IRS says we only have to hold our financial records for seven years. Why do we insist upon holding our emotional records for the rest of our lives?

Relational Healing

I've found that we can't see or live up to our full potential unless we are emotionally current, just as we can't be effective on the job if we spend the workday thinking about our unpaid debts. However, getting current with our emotional relationships is even more important than getting current with our bills. Actually, for most people, paying bills is *easy* compared to expressing feelings. Yet we've seen how important self-expression is in keeping the visual and energetic fields open. It's much harder to see clearly when we aren't expressing our feelings clearly. Some people even use poor vision as a way to avoid saying what they really feel—"out of sight, out of mind."

When we're emotionally clear, all of our senses are enhanced. We see freely and can share whatever we are seeing and feeling. Nothing is restraining either our eyes or our voice. How can we enhance our emotional self-expression and clear out the suppressed feelings that are at the root of our reluctance to express ourselves?

The other people in our lives may appear to be the source of our unresolved emotional issues, but what we think of as a problem with another person usually has very little to do with them. They are simply external mirrors of our inner experience. Everyone we meet in life offers us the opportunity to see ourselves more clearly—not just our partners, friends, and family but also our bosses, our coworkers, our enemies, our neighbors, and our casual acquaintances. We project our relationship with ourselves onto other people, just as we project our fear or anger onto the world as a visual blur.

I believe that we are innately social beings, and that relationships are the essence of life. Yet by restricting our vision, we are also restricting our ability to connect with others. Even after beginning the healing process, we may rely on inwardly oriented practices, such as meditation and visualization, to increase our self-awareness. Of course, these inner practices are invaluable tools for expanding awareness, but a growing self-awareness must eventually find an external expression in healthy relationships.

I believe that we cannot truly heal ourselves in isolation, and that integrating our full capacity for relationships—Relational Healing—is the most important aspect of any healing process. Reaching out to others sounds like a simple step, but it may actually be one of life's greatest challenges. Still, you'll find that if you make a firm intention to clear the blurred areas of your relationships, guidance and support will begin to come your way.

Unresolved emotions are usually the primary factor that keeps us from being fully present in our relationships. As you remove your lenses, you'll find that those previously suppressed feelings will spontaneously begin to arise and move. One of my colleagues described how she dealt with the feelings that began to surface after she reduced her prescription and wearing time:

> I made more space in my life—more time, more flexibility in my work and relationships. Because when those uncomfortable feelings came up, I needed to be able to let them move through me; I found that the opportunity for healing is only in the moment. And the feelings don't just come up when you're meditating, they come up throughout the day, at work, while you're shopping, anytime. To move through those emotions I used breathing and a willingness to feel my discomfort. Every time I let a big chunk of emotion move out, another level of my eyesight would clear up.

She makes a good point—it's much more difficult to move through your feelings when you don't have the time to hear what they're saying! Still, don't imagine that you have to quit your job and stop taking care of your family to get in touch with your feelings. Take a little more time for yourself and *be willing to notice* any feelings that come up, even when you're busy or distracted.

Keeping a Journal

To develop your ability to communicate feelings, you might want to begin keeping a personal journal. Science has now documented what many therapists have known for years: Spontaneous writing about our deepest feelings can be a very effective way to maintain emotional and physical health. Researchers have found that subjects who were "asked to 'write continuously without regard to spelling, grammar, sentence structure, etc.' on 'deeply personal topics' for '15–20 min[utes] a day for 3–5 consecutive days' [or more]" showed improved physical health (including "enhanced immune function"), better grades, fewer absentee days, and even "more success in finding a job."[1]

The "subjects who 'consistently expressed anxiety, sadness, and other words associated with negative feelings' were those who had 'the greatest improvements in physical health.'" Also, an increasing use of certain words—"understand," "realize," "because," "reason"—was found among those people with the greatest health benefits. The researchers determined that "the body expresses itself linguistically and biologically at the same time," and concluded that "writing . . . is a powerful therapeutic technique. Without instructions or feedback, subjects in our studies naturally [developed] common writing styles that promote physical and psychological health."

These people were asked to use the same technique therapists encourage: the keeping of a personal journal. This can be a surprisingly enjoyable way to increase self-understanding and to express emotions, especially when you're feeling overwhelmed. (If you've already begun to keep a vision journal, you can either expand it or start another notebook.)

This is how to start: Open your notebook, write the date and time at the top of the page, and begin to record whatever you are feeling. Some people like to write at the same time every day, but I suggest that you simply write whenever you feel the impulse. As you are writing, allow yourself to fully experience your emotions. Notice how your feelings shift as you record them, but don't try to analyze or justify anything. Just write down whatever you are feeling: "I'm scared. My heart is racing. My hands are sweaty. My breath feels stuck." Write spontaneously—don't worry about spelling or grammar! When you're done, put it away and forget about it. Don't go back and read it the next morning.

Writing in your journal is more than a way to express feelings and recenter yourself when you feel as if you're falling off a cliff. Every time you record an emotion, another one comes to the surface, and then another one. You are progressively emptying the bucket of fear within yourself.

Don't dwell on what you've written or reread it every day. Just get it off your chest. Someday, if you get a really strong impulse to review what you've been writing, pull out all your journals. Looking through them is like having a conversation with yourself. Choose a section that seems to be remote from your current concerns. As you read, notice how you've experienced the same feelings over and over. The awareness of those recurring emotions can be a revelation. We've seen how strong emotions—fear, hurt, anger—can lead to the collapse of the visual and energetic fields. And when those fields collapse, we lose our relationship with the past and the future. We can't remember what happened this morning, never mind last week.

Reviewing your journal is self-nurturing because it reflects the beauty of your true self back to you. As you see yourself more clearly, you develop deeper empathy and understanding of yourself. You begin to self-bond, to offer yourself the love and affection we all seek from others. You begin to realize how far you have come and can't help but pat yourself on the back: "What a great job you're doing. Congratulations!"

Love Letters

I've found that writing a series of "Love Letters" is also a very powerful tool for clearing out pent-up emotions that keep a person from being fully present. They can also be used to initiate communication and resolve conflict, but they are really about seeing and processing your own reflection. I first discovered the love letter format several years ago, through the work of John Gray, the author of *Men Are from Mars, Women Are from Venus.*

You'll need lots of paper or a notebook. On the first page, make a list of everyone with whom you have unfinished business. This can be either "good" business or "bad" business. Your list may include anyone you have strong feelings about, any relationship that has been "on your mind," any encounter that has left you feeling hurt or angry. Think through all your relationships: parents, children, friends, brothers and sisters, husbands, wives, ex-husbands, ex-wives, boyfriends, girlfriends, lovers, bosses and ex-bosses, coworkers, teachers, therapists . . . *anyone.* Don't forget to include yourself.

Look at the outline on the opposite page, "How to Write a Love Letter." This list of lead-in phrases takes you through an emotional progression from angry blaming to love. On a blank sheet of paper, write the name of whoever is on top of your list—for example, "Dear Mom." Write the first phrase, "I hate it when . . . ," and then put down everything that phrase brings to mind, everything about that person that you hate. "I hate it when you say . . . ," "I hate it when you do . . . ," "I hate it when you act like . . ." Keep writing until you have exhausted all of your "I hate it when . . ." feelings about that person.

Then go to the next phrase—"I don't like it when . . ."—and do the same thing. Keep writing until you have exhausted everything you can think of to say on that topic. Continue through each phrase on the list until you reach the end. You can add your own lead-in phrases to make sure that you feel complete with each of the five emotional stages. Sign the letter, "Love, (*your name*)," and date it. Then begin writing to the next person on your list.

Complete a letter to everyone on your list and put the letters away. Don't look at them or reread them; just put them away. In the

HOW TO WRITE A LOVE LETTER

Step One: ***Express Anger and Blame***
I hate it when...
I don't like it when...
I'm fed up with...

Step Two: ***Express Hurt and Sadness***
I feel sad when...
I feel hurt because...
I feel awful because...
I feel disappointed because...

Step Three: ***Express Fear and Insecurity***
I'm afraid that...
I feel scared because...

Step Four: ***Express Guilt and Responsibility***
I'm sorry that...
I'm sorry for...
Please forgive me for...
I didn't mean to...

Step Five: ***Express Love, Forgiveness,***
Understanding, and Hope
I love you because...
I love you when...
Thank you for...
I forgive you for...
I understand that...
I want...
I hope...

LOVE,

_____

meantime, you may have thought of other people to add to the list: "Oh, how could I have forgotten about Jim?" As these names come up, add them to the list and write them a letter. A few weeks after you have written the first letters write another set of letters to everyone on your list, without looking at the first letters. Just write down whatever comes to mind and date the letter. A few weeks after that, write another series of letters and date them. (The letters are really about you, not about anyone else. Normally you wouldn't show them to anyone unless you really felt that doing so would open a space for healing to occur.)

If you keep writing letters every few weeks, eventually you will sit down and find that you have nothing else to say. You won't hate anything, or be hurt by anything, or be afraid of anything about that person. All the unexpressed feelings will have been released from your system. When the only thing left to say is, "Dear ___ I love you because . . . ," you can consider yourself emotionally up to date in that relationship. That is the last love letter that you need to write to that person, and if you like, you can then have a little ceremony and burn all "their" letters!

Now that you've released those pent-up feelings, the next step is staying current. To do this, you must remain present with your feelings and express them to others as the need arises. When feelings come up, you'll share them with the other person—without blaming him or yourself. Then listen carefully, without interrupting, while he responds. If you have anything else to say, share that and continue the dialogue. You don't need to explain or justify why you feel what you are feeling, or expect the other person to do so either. Just keep sharing your feelings with each other as openly as you can.

This process has an incredible cleansing effect. Your relationships will become much richer as you recognize deeper levels of yourself in the mirror. Soon you will get to the point that when a feeling comes up, you won't want to wait even a moment to share it. You will want to go for it immediately. This feels both scary and wonderful.

As you get better at writing your feelings, you also get better at speaking them. If one day you again find yourself with feelings that you are afraid to share, sit down and write a letter before you talk to the other person. Allow your strongest feelings to come to the surface. After expressing your frustrations on paper, you'll be able to share in a much more responsible way. The steam will be out of your kettle. You will be able to express yourself honestly without dumping on or blaming the other person. You will be communicating from a much more balanced state.

You can also use love letters to resolve conflict. Show the other person how to write a love letter, and ask her not to leave out anything that is on her mind. Both of you write a love letter, then sit down and read your letters to each other. While one person reads, the other listens, without any interruptions or defenses—just listens. This very powerful exercise can clear the air for real love to come through.

Love letters are also a powerful technique to initiate and improve communication in families, groups, and organizations. Each person writes a letter to everyone else in the group. Then everyone sits down and reads their letters out loud to the group. In most groups, this brings to the surface so much pent-up emotion that you will probably want to have a neutral facilitator on hand!

Open Living

As you remove your glasses and begin to express your feelings, the limits of your perceptive field will begin to vibrate a little bit. After a while, the lock may come loose and a door may pop open. And the memories and feelings that have been hidden within you will begin to tumble out. At first, you may just notice that you feel different. Then one day, when you aren't looking for it, you may suddenly get a fresh inkling or a new piece of the puzzle. Usually you won't have any idea what it means yet.

Some time ago I was working with a woman—I'll call her Pamela—who told me that she was beginning to see the color red during our sessions, and she had no idea what it meant. She was having some issues with her mother, so I asked her mother to join us for a session. During our conversation, Pamela happened to mention that she was seeing red. Her mother looked startled, and then told us this story: "When Pam was about two years old, she accidentally locked herself in the laundry room. The door handle had broken a few weeks before, so my husband had turned the door around and hinged the other side. The door had been painted red, and now the red part was on the inside. Pam locked herself into that room with a red door. She couldn't get out and was screaming for help." As soon as Pamela heard that story, other memories began to surface—and she began to recall other traumatic experiences that she had been suppressing.

Pamela's experience is an example of what can happen as we begin to *see ourselves* again. Somehow we unlock a tiny fragment of our hidden self, and then one day it is revealed to be just one scene in a whole movie that we had forgotten. Then all of the emotions associated with that part of our life come rushing back into our awareness.

As long as we are suppressing those memories, the emotions associated with them can't flow through us, and our energy field eventually becomes as stuck as a sink with a clogged drain. Our senses become duller as the vital energy that moves our physical matter becomes stagnant. We may develop annoying physical symptoms or even become ill. By accessing and expressing those locked-in feelings, we can reopen our energy flow. This energetic release can have an immediate impact on our vision. For instance, as a young child, my daughter Gina used to tell me, "I always see better after I cry."

As our feelings begin to flow again, our life force returns to its natural power and our field expands. We may suddenly notice that our life feels too constricting. We may feel the need for a dramatic shift in our habitual attitudes and behavior.

As we keep our emotional channels open, we become more self-aware and develop healthier, more loving ways of relating to ourselves and others. Seeing effortlessly—Open Focus—may be the first step, but living effortlessly—Open Living—is our real goal. To reprogram ourselves for Open Living, we must access the body's own knowing, the *gut feelings* that, as Chopra says, "have not yet evolved to the level of self-doubt."[2] So in Part Three, I'll introduce you to a surprisingly enjoyable way to use that innate intelligence to rewire the body/mind for effortless living and seeing.

12 Vision Quest

By Rose Brandt, M.A.
Aspen, Colorado

I FIRST MET Jacob Liberman in Massachusetts in the spring of 1992. His book *Light: Medicine of the Future* had inspired a hope that I might someday be able to heal my vision the way he had. At the time, I'd worn strong lenses for myopia for about thirty years. My correction had progressed to around −6.00; my visual acuity was 20/800 in one eye and worse in the other—"off the chart," an eye doctor had once told me. I had no difficulty believing that vision improvement was possible—for other people. I was far from convinced that I could ever improve my own vision. In fact, it seemed like a hopeless dream. Nevertheless, I just couldn't get that "impossible" idea out of my head.

Jacob suggested a 20 percent reduction in my prescription and told me to wear even those glasses only when absolutely necessary. I took him very literally, so for the next month I didn't wear any lenses at all. This time was very frustrating, because I was expecting instant results and there didn't seem to be any noticeable improvement. Still, every time I was tempted to put my glasses back on, I would call Jacob and he would encourage me to look at my feelings instead. It was hard to look at the life-long backlog of painful feelings that were beginning to arise, but I was also feeling new energy to make some big changes in my life. I could already sense that clearing my vision would be just one aspect of a major process of self-transformation.

I moved to Colorado that fall, just in time to attend an intensive workshop that Jacob was giving in Aspen. His first words to us were a suggestion that we remove our glasses for the duration of the class. I hardly wore my glasses at all that week—and noticed a tremendous improvement in my vision. But it wasn't easy. I remember how scary it felt just to walk down an empty sidewalk without corrective lenses. The most frightening experience was when I walked into a grocery store. As I looked down the aisles, I was overcome by a feeling of panic. I felt blind, helpless, and cut off from the "real" world.

After the workshop I resumed wearing my weaker glasses part-time, since I needed them to see the computer screen while working. My vision got worse again, but even so, I passed the Colorado driver's test wearing the weaker lenses. Jacob rechecked my eyesight and said that I could reduce my prescription even further. Over the next year my vision seemed to fluctuate a lot, but I was able to gradually reduce my prescription a few more times. I found that my eyesight would improve whenever I went without lenses for a few days, and deteriorate whenever I wore a stronger pair, even for a few hours.

Shortly after I began to reduce my prescription, the regular migraines that I had had for years began to disappear—and within a few months they were gone. Now I get one only rarely. I used to think that they were inevitable and hereditary, but now I know they were related to wearing prescription lenses, because whenever I would put my glasses back on, all the muscles around my eyes, forehead, and temples would tighten up. It would be like trying to squeeze on a hat that's several sizes too small, which is just what my migraines felt like.

Since I often got a migraine after exposure to bright sunlight, I was quite hesitant when Jacob first suggested that I reduce my use of sunglasses. Still, I decided to try it anyway. I started using the sunning meditation (page 104) to adapt my eyes to brighter light, and it worked! I love to do sunning and still practice it regularly.

Within a few months, even the bright Colorado sun didn't bother me anymore, and I haven't worn any sunglasses since then.

Today my vision is still fluctuating and improving and often extremely clear. In the last few months my acuity has consistently been at least 20/40 whenever I have tried to read an eye chart. I still notice my blur indoors, but outdoors I can see with almost complete clarity.

Along the way there have been many breakthroughs, but I'll always remember my first experience of perfectly clear vision. It began as I was driving to Jacob's house one sunny day last summer. I was in the car practicing the blinking and tracing meditations (pages 99 to 100) when I suddenly realized that my vision was strikingly sharp, and that I was actually clearing it at will by blinking slowly and firmly. I'd always expected that I would be overjoyed to see clearly at last, but the intensity of my vision actually brought up a big surge of agitated fear, and I had to keep reclearing my eyesight.

When I arrived and told Jacob that I was seeing unusually well, he immediately got out an eye chart, paced off twenty feet (it looked like *fifty* feet to me), and held up the chart for me to read. The room was filled with glare and shadows, and the chart was backlit by the sun—I could hardly *see* the chart, never mind *read* it. I said, "Look, I can't see the chart where you're standing. Could you just step over into the light?" Jacob didn't move an inch but replied, "Just breathe and trace around the outline of whatever you *can* see." As soon as I began doing that, the entire chart popped into focus. He told me afterward that I had accurately read down to 20/25! That day my vision cleared up for the first time in over thirty years—and now that happens all the time.

However, my vision quest hasn't really been about learning to see more clearly. I can't say, for instance, that I have spent a lot of time doing the eye exercises. What I have focused on is the process of learning to be who I really am—of fully feeling all of the anger, fear, vulnerability, joy, and love that has been hidden within me. I understand now that my myopia was related to an inability to deal with the feelings involved in relationships. Despite lots of therapy, I could never really *feel* that issue while I was wearing glasses.

In the last year and a half, my world has changed dramatically. I've learned to stop struggling and enjoy life. I've learned more real and fulfilling ways of being in a relationship. I've learned to be much more patient and gentle with myself. In fact, I've gotten far more out of this process than I ever could have *dreamed* on the day I first removed my glasses.

PART
THREE

From Eyesight to Insight

13 Seeing the Invisible

*It is the commonest of mistakes to consider that
the limit of our power of perception is also the
limit of all there is to perceive.*
—*C. W. Leadbeater*

WE LIKE to assume that we see the world as it *really* is, that our eyes give us a full and accurate picture of reality. Yet physicists tell us that the visible world is simply an illusion *created by our senses,* that even the most "solid" objects are simply vibrational frequencies within a vast expanse of empty space. We know that vision is based on the perception of light, but what do we know about light? In the words of Albert Einstein, "Fifty years of . . . brooding have brought me no closer to the answer to the question, 'What are light quanta?' Of course today every rascal thinks he knows the answer, but he is deluding himself."[1]

The paradoxical nature of our perception of light is illustrated by an experiment conceived by the quantum physicist Arthur Zajonc, who designed a light box filled with a bright light that shone onto nothingness:

> We [took] special care to ensure that light [would] not illuminate any interior objects or surfaces in the box. Within the box, there is only pure light, and lots of it. The question is: What does one see? How does light look when left *entirely* to itself? . . .
>
> I look into the box and at the light within. What do I see? Absolute darkness! I see nothing but the blackness of empty space. . . . The space [is] . . . filled with light. Yet without an

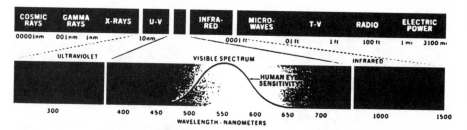

The Electromagnetic Spectrum (Reprinted with permission of General Electric Corporation, Lighting Division)

> object on which the light can fall, one sees only darkness. Light itself is always invisible. We see only things, only objects, not light.[2]

Not only is what we see *not* what we think it is, it is also an extremely small cross-section of the universe of electromagnetic energy that permeates our world. Our physical vision can only access a very limited frequency within the vastness of multidimensional reality—a tiny doorway called the "visible" portion of the electromagnetic spectrum (see the illustration above).

We usually assume that only modern technology can sense information carried on the television, radio, ultraviolet, infrared, microwave, or X ray frequencies. Yet I've found that as our field expands, we begin to perceive information that is supposed to be invisible to our normal senses. We "know" something before we are told, we "feel" the movement of invisible energy, or we "see" an event before it happens.

As our perceptive field expands, could it be drawing in a wider range of frequencies, just as a large radar screen can "see" farther than a smaller one? Could this extrasensory perception simply be our sensitivity to the invisible aspects of the electromagnetic spectrum, or even more subtle energy wavelengths as yet unknown to science? Some of our most prominent physicists have considered the possibility that there are forms of energy that science has yet to acknowledge:

> ALBERT EINSTEIN: "It is possible there exist human emanations that are still unknown to us. Do you remember how electrical

currents and 'unseen waves' were laughed at? The knowledge about man is still in infancy."

WERNER HEISENBERG: "Something has to be added to the laws of physics and chemistry before the biological phenomena can be completely understood."

People often comment on my "psychic" insights, but I've found that extrasensory facilities are a normal human ability that most of us have learned to suppress in childhood. Anyone can learn to see and feel the invisible; our inner or "psychic" vision emerges simultaneously as we expand the limits of our outer vision—as we open our eyesight, our psychic perception opens as well. Then we find that we are suddenly able to perceive far beyond the apparent limitations of our *physical* vision.

Remember Jacques Lusseyran, the French Resistance fighter who could see although his eyes had been destroyed? He warned sighted people "not to imagine that their way of knowing the world is the only one," and science is beginning to gather evidence that supports him. In a 1992 study, "invisible" ultraviolet (UV) radiation was found to produce visual responses in seven- to ten-year-old children. The researchers conclude that "the data presented here demonstrate that the perceptual capacities of some animals and young humans may be much broader than originally thought."[3] The researchers speculated that younger children would be able to see even farther into the UV range and that even adults would be able to perceive it to some extent.

In his book *Human Energy Systems,* the highly respected psychic Jack Schwarz describes an experiment at the University of Washington in which he was able to "see" energy well into the ultraviolet and infrared ranges—considerably above and below the "visible" portion of the electromagnetic spectrum. He feels that the only limits on our perception are those that are set by the mind, and that in certain states of consciousness our vision is unlimited. When he first began seeing the invisible he was told that he was hallucinating, seeing things that were not there. Yet when his "invisible vision" was being scientifically confirmed, other people who were tested were also able to see well beyond the normal range.[4]

Another "invisible" aspect of vision has to do with our assumption that seeing involves something *out there* that we bring inside our awareness to perceive and process. Vision is actually as much an emanation or projection of our awareness into the world as it is a perception of the outside world. As one researcher commented,

> The eye, like the hand ([or] the mouth), is an organ of manipulation, and . . . is . . . governed by the . . . brain. . . . It is the brain which [takes in] the outer world, whether manually, orally, or ocularly. It does so by a projective process, but this is a two-way, reciprocating process—a directional process which emanates from within the self, goes out, and then returns within.[5]

In the words of the physicist Karl Pribram, "Vision is a holographic projection." Energy (in the form of light) not only enters our sensory organs but actually emanates from them as our mind creates meaningful patterns from that input. This process is as yet not well understood, but in my experience it must be taken into account to get a full understanding of how vision really works. Vision seems to be not only a form of perception but also of self-expression or self-creation.

We think we know what vision is, and what it "looks" like. But as we move further into the realms of seeing the invisible, we find a form of intuitive sensing that has a very different appearance from physical eyesight. In most cases, psychics and sensitives will say they are "seeing" something, not "hearing" or "touching" it. Some nonphysical form of vision still seems to be the dominant way of receiving information. As we move past the boundaries of our normal eyesight, into the supposedly invisible portions of the electromagnetic spectrum (and possibly into as yet unknown forms of energy), vision as we know it seems to be transformed into a more global way of sensing, which may actually be the essence of *all* vision.

Seeing the Aura

One of the first "invisible" energies that you may begin to see is the *aura,* the part of the energy field that can be perceived as glowing light around the body. (Some people begin to see the aura almost spontaneously, while others may spend years learning to develop this ability.) The different colors of the aura are simply various light frequencies—wavelengths of light energy. It seems that the energetic frequencies that reach the earth's surface from the sun are perfectly balanced to support life on earth. I have found, however, that most of us only allow selected color frequencies to move fully through our system. The light that is able to move through us can be seen as the colors of the aura.

Jacques Lusseyran began to see auras only after his physical sight had been completely destroyed. Then "all the colors of the rainbow" began to return to his inner sight.

> My father and mother, the people I met or ran into in the street, all had their characteristic color which I had never seen before I went blind. Yet now this special attribute impressed itself on me as part of them as definitely as any impression created by a face.[6]

Some gifted psychics can see (or visualize) the aura while wearing corrective lenses, but I've found that the aura is very hard to see that way. Before removing my glasses, I had never seen an aura—in fact, I didn't even believe that auras were "real." I've now become convinced that in childhood we are all open to a wide range of extrasensory perception until we become socialized to conform to "normal" limitations.

The innocent extrasensory receptivity of children is well illustrated by a remarkable book, *The Boy Who Saw True*. It is the apparently authentic diary of a young boy in Victorian England, who spontaneously saw auras and just assumed that everyone else could, too. (The author did not want this revealing document to be released to the public during his lifetime, and it was first published in the 1950s.) On March 1, 1885, he complains that his parents refuse to answer his simple questions: "I asked mamma why her lights [aura] often went bluer when she was in church. And what do you think she said? She said to papa, 'I'm beginning to wonder if there isn't something wrong with that boy's eyes.' . . . Why wont mamma tell me things when I ask her? I would like to know why there is a lot of yellow like buttercups round papa's head and only blue round mother's, though sometimes when she hugs me very hard it goes pink. And I would like to know why Mildred's [his sister's] lights are just a mess like the [yolk] of a dirty egg."

Then the next day he reports, "I was let off lessons this morning because Mamma took me to town to see about my eyes. A funny little man in black made me look at a big card all covered with letters, and then he stuck up bits of glass I had to stare through. When I had been doing this for a long time, I heard him say to mamma, 'there is nothing to worry about, madam, the little gentleman has perfect sight.' "[7]

How much have we changed in the last hundred years? How many of us would know how to respond to this little boy's questions, other than to take him to an eye doctor?

A gifted clairvoyant (like the little boy above) can often see distinct colors and shapes emanating from the body. This ability seems to be inborn in all of us to some extent, and can be developed with practice. Auras are easier to see than you might think. Most people initially see the aura as a subtle white glow around the head. You might have already seen this effect and dismissed it as "visual fatigue" or by thinking that your eyes were playing tricks on you.

Although a full spectrum of white light enters each one of us, every aura is different, just as every face or set of fingerprints is unique. Since the aura only radiates the colors that are allowed to move freely through us, it is constantly shifting as we react to internal and external stimuli. As it moves, expanding and contracting, it is a constant barometer of our relationship to life in every moment.

Many healers and psychics can "read" a person's character, health, and state of awareness—even their entire life story—just by seeing (or "feeling") this energy field. Although he couldn't get any answers from his mother, the little boy in The Boy Who Saw True had already noticed that certain colors in the aura were associated with different personalities and feeling states. Many years later, he commented:

> I was at that time too inexperienced to know what the various colors indicated.[8] . . . I later on discovered that the type of aura I then described as "a dirty mess" denoted a complete

lack of emotional control, with little or no mentality, and that an aura with a hard outline was a sign of conventionality.[9]

Here's a simple practice to help you begin to see auras. Some people will notice striking effects right away, while others will need more patience. It can be helpful to keep reminding yourself that your awareness already knows how to perceive and read auras, just as your eyes already know how to see:

Practice on yourself by looking into a mirror that reflects a plain light-colored wall. Stand in front of the mirror and look toward your face but not at it, as in Open Focus. Or gaze just past the edges of your face—you may notice the aura in your peripheral vision. Either way, keep your eyes moving; don't stare at one spot.

As you do this, you may suddenly notice what looks like a glow of light or energy, but as soon as you turn your *focus* on it, it disappears! Practice observing whatever you're seeing without directly looking at it.

You can do this regularly, for as often and for as long as you like. Above all, don't discount or try to analyze anything you see or experience; simply allow yourself to be fully open to your own perception.

Barbara Ann Brennan is a well-known clairvoyant and energy healer. In her book *Hands of Light,* she describes how she discovered that her auric vision could be used to rebalance the body/mind and initiate healing:

> I was rather skeptical when I first started "seeing" the energy phenomena around people's bodies. But since the phenomena persisted, even if I closed my eyes to make it go away or moved around the room, I began to observe it more closely . . . I saw that the energy field is intimately associated with a person's health and well-being. . . . [By reading the energy field] I have become proficient in diagnosing both physical and psychological problems and in finding ways to resolve those problems. . . . [10]

How does the light of the aura reflect our being so clearly? We can compare this process to a glass prism (see the figure on page 166).

When white light, which contains all visible wavelengths of color, enters one side of a prism, the individual colors are separated, and

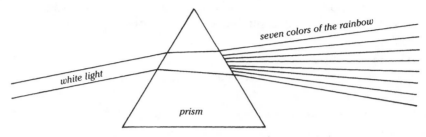

Light Passing Through a Prism

a rainbow of color is emitted from the other side. The prism does not block or hold on to any aspect of the light, so the full spectrum passes through the prism with all its colors intact. Yet I've never seen a rainbow emanating from a human being. Our areas of emotional and energetic contraction usually block all but a few light frequencies from flowing freely through our system. I've never seen anyone clear enough to radiate a rainbow.

Also, it appears that when we *are* able to emanate all colors, they don't remain separate, as in a prism, but merge again into white light. We know that artists have traditionally depicted great saints as surrounded by a bright halo of light or energy. I used to think that the halo was just an artistic convention, but it is no coincidence that holiness is so often shown this way. Throughout history there have been many reports of holy people who radiated a brilliant light that could be seen by anyone around them.

It seems that when sunlight enters the field of an enlightened one, it meets no resistance or attachment. All the colors of the rainbow merge and radiate outward in a full spectrum of dazzling white light. The auras of these saints are so clear and bright that they are even visible to the average person's limited sight. In his wonderful book *The Holographic Universe,* Michael Talbot relates some examples:

> Many cultures believe that the aura of an extremely spiritual individual is so bright it is visible even to normal human perception, which is why so many traditions, including Christian, Chinese, Japanese, Tibetan, and Egyptian, depict saints as having halos or other circular symbols around their heads. In his book on miracles Thurston[11] devotes an entire chapter to

accounts of luminous phenomena associated with Catholic saints, and both Neumann and Sai Baba are reported to have occasionally had visible auras of light around them. The great Sufi mystic Hazrat Inayat Khan . . . is said to have sometimes given off so much light that people could actually read by it.[12]

Any contraction in our field (such as occurs when we become afraid or tense) blocks some aspect of light energy as well as our receptivity to certain emotions or experiences. Those aspects of life then become invisible to us, just as we blur out areas of perception when we become nearsighted or farsighted. Clearing our physical vision eventually brings us to the point where we begin to see and emanate more of those invisible areas of life. We begin to feel more whole, less fragmented, more fully ourselves.

My own inner vision began to reawaken shortly after the meditative experience that I called "becoming the sky." That year I went on a Caribbean vacation and took a ride on a large boat. I was relaxing at the back of the boat, just enjoying my Open Focus, when suddenly I started seeing what looked like halos around the other people. At first I thought it was just the light playing tricks on my eyes. When it didn't go away, I panicked, thinking that I must have had a retinal detachment. I wanted to go straight to an eye doctor. But there was nothing wrong with my eyes. It was simply my first experience of seeing the light emanating from the human energy field.

Quantum Vision

When you look at an ambient background, such as a blue sky or a white wall, you can sometimes see shiny little particles flickering in the air. Medical textbooks call this phenomenon *Muscae Volitantes,* and explain it as light reflecting off the cells in the eye:

> *Muscae Volitantes:* This term is employed for the appearance of spots (motes) before the eyes. . . . They are caused by the shadows cast upon the retina by the cells normally found in the vitreous humor or by tiny developmental remnants, and occur in all eyes, being seen in certain conditions such as exposure to a uniform bright surface. . . . They are annoying and sometimes alarm the patient, but are of no importance. . . .

They persist and annoy the patient until he ceases to look for them and thus forgets their existence.[13]

That physiological explanation may be correct, as far as it goes, but I believe that there is more to it than that. Sometimes it seems that we are actually seeing into the vibrational essence of material reality. If "solid" objects are really composed of vibratory waves in empty space, how can we be so sure we cannot perceive this energy?

One explorer of consciousness (a saint who was simply known as "Mother") wrote that she fell into a "vastness . . . made of countless imperceptible dots—dots that take up no space—of a warm, dark gold. All that was absolutely alive, alive with a power that seemed infinite. And yet motionless. A perfect immobility, but containing an incredible intensity of movement and life! . . . It was like a powdering . . . a multitude of tiny gold dots, nothing but that." Her biographer commented that she "had emerged at the atomic level, that her body *was living* quantum physics."[14]

Maybe Jack Schwarz was right; maybe we *can* see more than we think we can. For instance, we assume that the air around us is invisible—but is it? When you look at an ambient background, there is nothing to focus on and you may spontaneously shift into Open Focus. Open Focus can reveal a whole new world of dynamic energy. When I started opening my focus to see the entire visual field, I began to see dazzling, swirling energy configurations everywhere I looked.

Most people can perceive this "invisible" energy, but usually we ignore it. You might like to try this experiment: If you're wearing glasses or contacts, take them off. Now look softly toward an ambient background, such as a blank wall, and open your focus so that your eyes are moving spontaneously and you are seeing everything in your visual field with equal clarity. As your eyes wander freely, notice anything that you see "in the air"—look *into* the air instead of *past* it. You may become aware of a kind of moving texture or soft shimmering. Allow your eyes to follow this shimmer for a while. Some of the effect may appear to originate within your eyes, and some of it may appear to be in the air. You may also notice subtle wave-forms that seem to have no definite location.

This observation has allowed you to see a perfectly visible aspect of reality that is normally invisible, just because our central focus—the aspect of our mind's eye that looks hard—tends to look past it or through it. Wearing corrective lenses will also close off that aspect of our vision. That's why many people who have spent time without glasses notice how "flat" and "empty" their vision seems whenever they put their glasses back on.

In Open Focus, the whole world sparkles and resonates with life. This shimmer seems to be a vital energy that surrounds and permeates everything, even "empty space." Could this vibrant energy be an aspect of the quantum reality that composes everything in the Universe? It does appear to be the same energy that composes our auras and energy fields.

I've found that most people can learn to see or sense auras and invisible energy by practicing Open Focus. However, as soon as we try to analyze this new vision, our ability to see the invisible temporarily disappears. It seems to be based on a specific state of mind, a meditative awareness. As soon as we try to figure out how we are doing it, it's gone. By looking for proof or evidence, we have moved into a discriminating mode and out of Open Focus.

We have learned to ignore or dismiss much of the information coming in through our "normal" channels, never mind from our extrasensory perception. Every time we suppress the evidence of our senses, their sensitivity diminishes. As we remove our lenses, clear our vision, and learn to see the invisible, we simply reverse that process. We return our awareness to the information that we have previously dismissed because it didn't fit our concepts about reality. Here is an exercise to enhance that sensitivity:

Begin to practice Open Focus whenever you are looking at people, animals, or plants. Notice how the invisible energy swirls around them, just as it did against the blank wall in the previous exercise. Notice where your eyes are drawn and any impressions that enter your awareness. Are your eyes trying to tell you something about this person? Do you sense that their energy is open or blocked in certain areas?

Above all, don't discount or try to analyze anything you see or experience. Simply allow yourself to be fully open to your own perception.

As you remove your lenses and practice the suggestions given in Part Two, you'll find that seeing details more clearly is only a small aspect of the benefits you'll receive. For instance, as your ability to see the invisible expands, your "dream vision" may begin to shift. Even if you don't usually remember your dreams, you may begin to remember dream images that are clearer and more colorful than ever before. A woman who for several months had been reducing her prescription and wearing time had this dream experience:

> My vision is weakest in the dark, and I still use my contacts for night driving. Yet in this dream I was driving on a very dark night, and I could see everything with *perfect* clarity. This was a very vivid experience and I wondered how I was seeing so clearly, because I knew I wasn't wearing my lenses. I kept trying to understand it. Then it struck me very strongly that this was my real vision—that I really *could* see this clearly, *if only I would let go of my "habit" of myopia.* I awoke with the powerful feeling that I had had a profound breakthrough in understanding and clearing my vision.

This dream illustrates the deeper level of understanding that we begin to access as our receptive field opens up. With this greater sensitivity we may begin to understand the possibility of psychic healing or perceiving the future, to name just two activities that involve *seeing the invisible.* In fact, I've found that the more we open up, the more we realize that our nature is to continuously expand our range of possibilities. It really seems that nothing is truly "impossible." We simply set our mental boundaries of "possibility" in a certain position and then move them around as our awareness shifts.

Working with Invisible Energy

After confirming that I didn't have a retinal detachment, I began to investigate my experience on the boat more deeply, and I realized that I had begun seeing auras. From then on I started to see auras more and more frequently. This was an exciting area that I knew very little about, so I decided to experiment by observing my clients' auras as I worked with them. I had no idea what I would find. I simply began to notice and share whatever I was seeing. Eventually I realized that simply "reading" the aura was actually limiting the information I could receive.

Our eyes are designed to tune into anything that is out of place in our perceptive field. Since the life force within us and around us is in constant motion, "out of place" often means stagnant, stuck energy. Thinking hard and blocking feelings are the most common causes of stagnant energy. These patterns seem to place little dams across the river of our awareness, around which our vital flow has to work its way. This circuitous process creates a lot of unnecessary struggle and effort, so these habitual energetic blockages often eventually manifest as emotional or physical symptoms.

My ability to see invisible energies seemed to be expanding far beyond reading the aura. My eyes were being automatically drawn to any place in the energy field where the person's energy felt blocked or stuck. This is still how I usually perceive the energy field: a "seeing feeling" or an "intuitive sensing" that is often accompanied by a symbolic image.

Sometimes I just receive the image, without a sense of its meaning, but usually the image is a therapeutic doorway that has a clear significance to either myself or the client. The person might appear to have an arrow through his chest, or some part of his body might appear to be empty or caved in. Whatever the image, when I describe it the client usually responds, "Yes, that's exactly what's going on there," or "That's just what it feels like."

When I first started getting these images, seventeen or eighteen years ago, I thought, This is ridiculous! I remember the first time I had the courage to share what I was seeing. I was still practicing optometry at the time and was doing an eye exam on a woman in my office. For some reason my attention kept getting drawn to her throat, like an artist being drawn to the part of a painting that still needs some work. Something in her throat appeared to be dark or stuck, and I didn't understand it.

After the exam was over I felt I just had to ask her what was going on in her throat. She started crying, and said, "How did you know?" She said that she had had thyroid surgery and was on thyroid medication. She also felt that her throat represented a deep, unresolved emotional issue with her mother, which had preceded her thyroid problem. As she was telling me this, I saw an image of a bird flying out of a cage. I sensed that whatever had been trapped inside her throat had been released.

Assisting the flow of invisible energy is now the most powerful aspect of my energetic work. Often when I'm working on someone in a group, others may also see the energy exchange taking place. Here's what one participant told me she saw as I was working with a woman I'll call Jane: "The first thing that caught my attention was when I suddenly started to see Jane's immense aura, a very wide, kind of cloudy white aura, and also your hands and arms in a beautiful turquoise green light moving around her. It was like the green color that surgeons wear to operate—it looked as if I could only see Jane's aura and a pair of green gloves flying, moving in the air around her."

We are all meant to sense that invisible energy, but it is rarely perceptible as long as we are wearing corrective lenses. The first step in developing the ability to work with energy fields is to remove your lenses! Then simply notice what you see and begin to share those perceptions with others.

When I first began to observe my clients' auras, I just noticed that they were constantly fluctuating. Then I began to notice that certain fluctuations were associated with specific states of mind and visual changes. One day I realized that every time a person would start to think hard or analyze, his aura would shrink to the point that it would almost disappear! At the same time, his vision might suddenly blur as well.

This was a shock. I had already become convinced that the aura was a mirror of the state of the energy field, as the ancient seers had taught. If the aura shrinks every time we concentrate our thoughts, then the perceptive and expressive capacity of our field must also shrink every time we think! I began to wonder what could be going on in the mind to create this disturbing effect. After all, I had been taught that logical thought was the pinnacle of evolution, the primary element that separated humans from the animals. How could it be detrimental to the flow of our vital energy?

14 The Truth About Thinking

*It seems that I have spent my entire time trying to make
life more rational and that it was all wasted effort.*
—A. J. Ayer

I HAVE FOUND that the most common addiction in the world does
not involve drugs, cigarettes, or alcohol; it occurs whenever we go
into our thoughts to avoid our feelings. We may not even realize we
are doing it, but thinking hard is one of the easiest ways to shut off
any discomfort, fear, or pain—as well as vision. We've learned to
take thinking for granted; it pervades every aspect of our lives, and
we further reinforce its dominance by wearing corrective lenses. We
believe we need to think ahead, pay attention, make plans in order
to achieve our goals. However, most of that planning and thinking
simply distracts us from whatever we are experiencing *now,* which
is the source of our spontaneous knowing and intelligence.

What exactly do we mean by "thinking" or "the mind"? We've come
to use these terms to describe every aspect of our ability to know,
perceive, analyze, or discriminate. But defining all these dissimilar
states of mind as "thinking" is misleading. I have noticed two fundamental types of perception that appear to be related to two very different aspects of the mind. You could call them two categories of
knowing: hard (or narrow) thinking and effortless (or open) thinking.

These two ways of thinking reflect our two ways of seeing: looking hard (tunnel vision), which occurs as the field contracts, and
looking effortlessly (Open Focus), which occurs as the field ex-

pands. In fact, how we think actually seems to determine how we see—as might be inferred from the physiological link between the eyes and the brain. Further confirmation comes from the work of the behavioral psychologist Marcel Just, who studied how the pupil of the eye responds to the intensity of thought. His research revealed that "the eye [is] a kind of meter of mental energy."[1]

To understand how we see, we must examine how we think—and changing our habitual way of thinking can improve our chronic vision difficulties. A large part of this mental/visual shift occurs spontaneously as we remove or reduce the strength of our lenses, but we can help it along by understanding what is happening. Then healing can occur simultaneously in both the eyes and the mind—as you help your eyes become more whole, you help your mind become more whole, and vice versa. Dr. Bates noticed this connection many years ago: "You can teach people how to produce any error of refraction, how to produce a [crossed eye], how to see two images of an object . . . at any angle from each other, simply by teaching them how to think in a particular way."[2] Visual problems can also be alleviated, as well as induced, through the mind.

The most common mental pattern in our culture is thinking *hard.* This is how we process linear information, like arithmetic, and logical relationships, such as cause and effect. Since we are thinking hard whenever we are discriminating, analyzing, or judging, hard thinking has been the basis for almost all modern science and technology. It is associated with our central vision, which focuses beautifully but cannot hold the vision of the whole. Because it is the focusing aspect of our mind (and our vision), thinking hard tends to be reinforced whenever we try to concentrate or become afraid.

Fear is a powerful concentrator of our attention, and the shift from effortless thinking (feeling connected) to hard thinking (feeling separated) is usually related to fear. Fear is simply a natural response, like other emotions. It is only when we are afraid to feel fear that we become stuck in it. Instead, we go into our thoughts to distract ourselves from it. As our attention narrows, the natural rhythm of our energy field—its continuous expansion and contraction—goes into spasm and we lose some of our openness and flexibility.

Analytical thinking is the dominant state of mind in modern society, but the analytical mind is unable to feel, because feeling is a global, rather than a linear, function. The result is that most people nowadays can't think and feel simultaneously. Yet when we think without feeling we can perceive and process so little of our total experience! Thinking hard is the habitual mental state of a narrow mind, tunnel vision, or a closed field of awareness. When we think with effort, we are not aware of the full range of our knowledge, perception, or understanding, because we lose sight of the whole. We only seem to be able to access a tiny fragment of our mind, which I call the local mind, because it seems to be confined to our brain or our head.

Seeing and thinking in this focused way plays an important role in our lives; the problem is that we have come to rely on it almost exclusively. As Albert Einstein remarked, "The problems we have cannot be solved at the same level of thinking we were at when we created them." We have forgotten that there is another, equally important, way to view the world. We have come to believe that the only valid way to think is to contract our awareness to the point where we lose sight of the whole.

Dr. Sampooran Singh, who has researched the human mind-brain system, also believes that we must now move toward balance by enhancing our capacity for *global* or *open* thinking:

> Many eminent scientists—including Einstein, Heisenberg, Shrödinger . . . have stumbled upon another mode of knowing, called intimate, direct, intuitive, insight, non-dual knowledge. . . .
>
> Humanity now needs to go beyond the analytical, fragmented mind, always dissecting, comparing, evaluating, to another kind of perception—which is direct understanding of life or insight and intuitive awareness of the true nature of life.[3]

Open thinking transcends our familiar local mind and linear processing to access the intelligence of the nonlocal mind, the greater hologram. Whole intelligence is a very different experience from linear thought—in the first place, it can *feel*. It has "the capacity to understand life directly, or to perceive intuition, or to perceive the wholeness of life. [It] keeps alive the spiritual intuition. The perception of wholeness conveys the world of meaning and values, a new ethical outlook."[4]

Linear thinking tries to separate thought from other ways of knowing (such as impulses, feelings, and intuitions) in an attempt to discriminate more clearly. Whole intelligence, however, unifies all those sources of insight into one "holistic knowledge experience." In this state, thoughts and ideas arise spontaneously from gut feelings, just as the neuropeptides within our cells do. Discrimination still occurs, as a form of effortless knowing originating at a higher level of perception than the local mind can access.

In our dreams we usually perceive and think holographically—in terms of wholes. Instead of having one thought or event logically follow another, many dreams seem to consist of overlapping wholes of thoughts, feelings, and events. This is why some dreams are very difficult for our linear mind to unravel after we wake up. Unless there is a distinct story line, our linear mind tries to impose order onto what feels like a chaotic dream memory. Even in "story" dreams, we may simultaneously play a role in several parallel story lines. We may awake from such a dream feeling disappointed because the holographic dream awareness feels so much deeper and richer than our ordinary (linear) awareness.

We can find other examples of holographic thinking in recent research on out-of-body experiences (OBEs) and near-death experiences (NDEs). Although usually still dismissed by mainstream science, the increasingly sophisticated research in these areas actually provides us with a very clear and consistent picture of how holographic thinking operates. Robert Monroe, the author of *Journeys Out of the Body* and *Far Journeys,* and founder of a pioneering research institute on OBEs, reports that holographic thought is *the* method of communication used in OBEs. He refers to it as "thought balls" or NVC (nonverbal communication):

> [NVC] is something far more than what we label body language, telepathy, remote viewing, [etc.]. We say that a picture is worth 1,000 words. A color picture is worth 10,000 words. A moving color picture is worth 50,000 words, perhaps, and a talking moving picture is worth 100,000 or more words in the transmission of information and/or communication.

> NVC takes a quantum jump beyond a talking moving color
> picture. It is direct instant experience and/or immediate know-
> ing transmitted from one intelligent energy system and
> received by another.[5]

Writing about near-death experiences, Michael Talbot confirms
Monroe's description: "Individuals . . . in [the near-death] realm . . .
communicate through a telepathic series of 'light pictures.' "[6]

There seems to be a universal hologram, the greatest whole that
our minds can conceive of, which is the ultimate source of intelligence, of knowing. I believe that this universal awareness is constantly radiating information, the way the sun radiates energy.
When our field is open, we receive that information intuitively as a
whole "information packet" or "thought ball," which spontaneously
stimulates a whole response—from the gut. Another way of saying this is that when our field is open, we never have to think
to know. The spontaneous flow of receptivity and response
requires no linear processing. In fact, thinking hard will instantly
cut it off. In comparison, linear thought appears shallow and
almost mechanical.

We usually assume that thinking means concentration, but
thought requires no more intentional focusing than vision. In fact,
we may be able to process the most complex levels of information
only by allowing our thoughts to flow organically and effortlessly.
This flow of knowing characterizes artistic creativity and genius in
all fields, so why do we tend to assume that open thinking is any
less intelligent than hard thinking?

In open thinking, we leave behind almost all of our fixed beliefs,
expectations, and judgments. In fact, in comparison to thinking hard,
it almost feels as if we have no mind. We are so used to the narrow
blinders of our local mind that we don't realize how much they block
our perception. In open thinking, our awareness feels effortless and
unlimited, as if we are accessing the infinite mind of God.

The mental process of open thinking parallels the visual process
of Open Focus. We can begin to think effortlessly anytime we enter
Open Focus, or whenever we simply become fully present. Then we
can discover through our own experience that our mind requires no
more direction or control than our eyes. Another powerful doorway

to opening our mind is movement (which is covered in detail in the last few chapters).

We believe that linear thinking is the great evolutionary leap that has placed us "in control" of life on earth—but what do we really think about most of the time? Usually, we are simply worrying, trying to stay "in control" by thinking in obsessive circles like a hamster on a wheel. Worrying and thinking hard are simply indicators that we don't feel safe enough to trust the instinctive wisdom of our belly brain, which leads to a chronic internal rehearsal of our life.

I often hear people say, "I'm confused." What does that mean? Is there really any such thing as "confusion"? When we start to think, our awareness shrinks. We're too anxious to think clearly, and we're thinking too hard to feel how anxious we are. Then we may say, "I'm confused." If we say that often enough, we may begin to believe it's true. However, all that is usually happening is that our thoughts are so active that we can't feel our feelings. We may also say, "I'm confused" when we know what we see or want to do but are afraid to see or do it!

When that happens, we can't make a move or a decision without sending the impulse "up to committee," where it is endlessly argued back and forth. We compare the present to our limited memory of the past and project it into the future. We forget that there's no way to achieve full resolution of our "confusion" without accessing the wisdom of the whole *in the present.* This is how we often keep ourselves locked into doubt and confusion.

Toward the end of his life, the "visionary physicist" David Bohm began to focus on the problem of thinking:

> Thought, he proposed, is the devil that got us into the present crisis. Thought designed our unworkable institutions. Because thought gets no immediate feedback from the physical world, it is truly a loose cannon.
>
> Consider: If we're learning to walk . . . we get immediate and ruthless feedback. We slip, spill, bump, fall . . . and we learn. Yet there is no counterpart of this immediate feedback for an errant thought. As we mature we can pick up [a] teacup skillfully, but we have no way of knowing whether our beliefs hold water. Our thinking can be off the wall and often is, but our brains don't say "ouch!" or "missed it!"[7]

We may not get immediate feedback, but unfortunately we have now created an entire world that reflects the mistaken belief that we can only learn, succeed, and be loved by others through thinking hard. That belief has created a vicious spiral of hard thinking, since it reinforces the idea that life is a constant struggle. Whenever we think hard, we restrict the breath that carries the life force, subtly fragmenting our body/mind. We end up with a world full of problems caused by living in our heads while holding our breath.

When we think hard, we break our relationship to ourselves, as well as to the outside world. We constrict our breath, shut out our spontaneous wisdom, shrink our energy field, and segment our awareness. As we lose the ability to access our effortless knowing, we can't learn easily or see clearly. We become separate from the world, separate from others, and separate from ourselves.

I used to attend many optometric conferences and sit in on the presentations. I never could understand what was going on: They would shut off all the lights, project a series of slides onto a screen, and fill our heads with statistics. Some people in the audience would fall asleep, while others would just sit quietly, pretending not to be bored. I kept wondering, "Don't those doctors realize that *they* are the remedy, not their information?" We got the information, but we never got the real message—their presence. The presentations never stayed with me afterward; they would go in one ear and out the other without stopping. My body/mind hadn't heard anything worth remembering.

I remembered the same dilemma from grade school. Although I had tried to "pay attention," I had instinctively known that the lessons were unrelated to my real needs and interests. Later I worked in grade schools as a developmental vision consultant. I noticed that since children have less-developed linear thinking skills than adults, if their whole self isn't engaged in the learning process they just get bored. I was working with children who had various kinds of visual problems, and most of them were also classified as "learning disabled" in some way. I began to wonder whether the epidemic of visual and learning problems in our schools could be related to the way we encourage children to think.

15 Effortless Seeing, Effortless Learning

It is as natural for the eye to see as it is for the mind to acquire knowledge, and any effort in either case not only is useless but defeats the end in view.
—Dr. William Bates

LIKE THINKING, the ability to learn is intimately connected to how we see: 90 percent of what we learn is taken in by our vision. Anything that influences how we process visual information will affect our learning potential. Most people don't realize that seeing clearly is just one of many vision skills required for reading and learning. Developmental optometrists have found that "80 percent of 'slow' readers (. . . children two or more grade levels behind in reading) experience difficulty in control and coordination of the eyes."[1] And "children with difficulty controlling and coordinating their eyes are often above average in [visual] acuity. 'They'd make great buffalo hunters, but often are not good students.' "[2]

The other skills necessary for learning include "the ability to track, focus and coordinate the eyes together as a team, [as well as] visual discrimination, form perception, visual memory and the integration of visual information with other sensory systems."[3] In fact, one eye doctor lists *twenty* visual skills that are required in order to read without stress.

Unfortunately, many of these essential skills are not tested in the standard eye exam and so most cases of visually related learning problems are never discovered. Yet their eventual effects can be quite serious, as the child who cannot read without significant visual stress often becomes defeated and disillusioned: "Parents and teachers often label kids as dumb, lazy, unmotivated, looking for attention, or as poor students, when what is really wrong is that they have undetected vision problems. They become dropouts—not only from school but from a full life."[4]

Deficient visual skills often lead to low self-esteem and difficulty in coping with life in general: "Failure in reading . . . generalizes to failure in school (80 percent of school work depends on good reading skills) and eventually in . . . illiteracy . . . increased dropout [rate], drug usage and delinquency."[5] Dr. Stanley Kaseno, a vision therapist who has worked extensively with juvenile delinquents, says that "we find an absolute correlation between vision disorders, reading disabilities and juvenile delinquency. [And no intervention] program works well without the youngster's ability to learn and think problematically."[6]

But effective and relatively inexpensive treatment *is* available. In fact, Ray Gottlieb estimates that "90 percent of . . . vision problems associated with reading can be alleviated."[7] Visually related learning disorders are treated by optometric vision therapy, which is practiced by behavioral optometrists, among others. Vision therapy is based on the link between how we see and how we think: "When your eyes are examined . . . by the optometrist who practices vision therapy, it is quite literally an examination of the way your brain functions. . . . [The optometrist is] in effect working with the brain, the body's central control."[8] Another eye doctor describes vision therapy as "a type of intellectual training, of the most vital order."[9]

Vision therapy can affect far more than our learning skills: "New patterns of eye movement can translate into a more fluent way of being in the world, just as habitual patterns of visual strain and overvigilance turn into psychological and body tension."[10]

In fact, visually related learning problems really begin in the mind, at the level of our awareness—*awareness* seems to be the underlying source of learning problems, just as it is for vision problems. Our way of seeing is only the mirror of our way of thinking, attending, and processing information. When we develop a gap or warp in our awareness, that break is transmitted to our vision, which interferes with our ability to receive new information, creating a vicious cycle of perceptive and cognitive difficulties. Both vision and learning problems begin at a far more basic level than the visual system, and we can most effectively transform them by accessing their source in our awareness.

Paying Attention

We can vividly see the effects of hard thinking in the elementary school classroom. When they start school, most children still express themselves freely. But as they discover that to be loved and rewarded they must *try to learn* and *think before they speak,* they tend to become fragmented thinkers, hesitant readers, and even stammering speakers. Children quickly learn that they will be recognized and acknowledged not for whole thinking but for separating their mind from their intuitions and segmenting their holistic perception into "pieces of knowledge."

Stuttering is an extreme example of this fragmentation. I've worked with many children who stutter. It's interesting: They don't stutter when they are singing or when they are moving and breathing freely. At first I wondered why. Then I realized that they couldn't think *hard* while doing these whole-brain activities. Vocal stuttering seems to be a reflection of stuttering by the entire awareness, a constant interruption in our relationship to the world.

We were taught to learn by "paying attention," but as we strain to think hard, our field collapses and our vision contracts. A shrunken field can only process incoming information like a tape recorder, by recording it and playing it back. We can't really absorb new information unless our perceptive field is relaxed and open. I began to wonder how we could maintain an expanded state of awareness while learning.

One of the biggest misconceptions about thinking, seeing, and learning is that they require effort to function at their best. We've already seen how effort actually reduces our visual clarity and limits our intelligence—and this also applies to learning. Children spontaneously know how to think globally and learn effortlessly. They simply need to be allowed to use these inborn abilities. Each of us seems to be designed to absorb certain subjects like a sponge. We may be bored to tears by other topics, especially when they are taught as unintegrated pieces of linear information that seem to have little relevance to our own experience.

Our educational system tries to conform children's minds to a standardized learning process (just as eye doctors "correct" our vision to the norm). It denies children's need to discover their own meaning and purpose. When you consider that children are also taught that they must compete for success and attention, it is no wonder that school is such a source of stress for so many of them. That frustration leads to low self-esteem and a constriction of the field, which can lead to both learning and visual problems.

Ray Gottlieb also believes that "a major cause of nearsightedness and other visual problems is the tension generated by current methods of education." He described how this occurs in an interview in the *Brain/Mind Bulletin:*

> Emphasizing the acquisition of information encourages excessive concentration, he said. "In school we are taught to squeeze and hold on to information—to be sure we've 'got it'— rather than let it come to us."
>
> As a result we learn to constrict our breathing, heartbeat and other physical movement—even blinking—in order to concentrate. . . .
>
> The educational system, he said, discourages or ignores what should be the first step in learning—self-awareness. . . .
>
> When Gottlieb asks young patients to "count to 10 and clap your hands on the number 5," many have no awareness of whether they performed the act correctly. "They often answer, 'I don't know—you tell me,' as if it is not their business to know such things."[11]

Several studies have confirmed the influence of school stress in triggering myopia, but this effect can also be reversed: One researcher documented "a very significant *decrease* in myopia in an elementary school program designed to reduce stress and anxiety."[12]

I'm often asked, "Isn't a certain amount of hard thinking *neces-*

sary in school to learn math and reading?" I don't think so. We sometimes forget that the miracles of life are not limited to flowers and animals. Humans are also meant to grow and develop spontaneously. According to a model of brain function developed by psychiatrist William Gray and systems scientist Paul LaViolette, "The brain uses feelings to structure information. A felt sense underlies everything we know. . . . When we are cut off from our feeling tones, mental connections become difficult. That is why abstract information is so hard to recall. . . . "[13] This model, which has been supported by several research studies, confirms that the best way to process *any* new information is open thinking, which allows us to access both thoughts and feelings simultaneously.

Children know that learning is meant to be as effortless as playing. Real learning is a deeply satisfying, joyful, magical experience, but many of us can't remember ever feeling the joy of learning. We usually think of learning as a purely mental task directed by an authority figure, a teacher, but that kind of learning goes in one ear and out the other. When we cram the mind with facts in order to take a test, by the next day we have forgotten most of what we worked so hard to memorize. However, when you're inspired by a great teacher, learning becomes as easy as falling in love, and what you learn through experience, you learn by heart. It becomes a part of who you are in every moment.

Effortless Learning

What is the key to effortless learning? Experience seems to be the most effective way to absorb new information. As Tim Gallwey, the author of *The Inner Game of Tennis,* has said, "One's own experience is the only real teacher. Effectively teaching others consists of making them more aware of *their experience,* not someone else's."[14]

Movement also seems to be how we program the meaning of new experiences into our awareness. "A shift of belief demands a shift in movement," according to "movement psychologist" Stuart Heller. "It is not enough to work on *either* the body *or* the mind. . . . Changing one's thinking typically makes no difference to the body.

Likewise, releasing physical tensions doesn't affect underlying beliefs. But you can affect both by directly altering the movement pattern that connects them."[15]

Unless we translate a new insight into body knowledge, it cannot be fully integrated into our awareness. Michael Gelb, the author of *Body Learning*, notes that "the first step in learning often is *un*learning what we know. The long-term effects of faulty body use cause wrong habits to feel right. We need to stop doing habitual things so that a natural mind/body coordination can emerge."[16] If that is true, then we might be able to reprogram the entire body/mind by retraining a person's habitual way of moving. Maybe effortless movement would lead to effortless seeing and effortless learning.

After all these years, *can* we acquire a different way to think and to learn? Yes. I've spent years developing a movement process that I call *Effortless Learning.* I've found it to be a very powerful healing tool not only for improving vision but also for limited awareness, narrow thinking, and learning difficulties of all kinds. It is based on the principle that when we learn through movement, we learn holographically rather than through the linear mind. During Effortless Learning, we can actually experience how our habitually narrow thinking repeatedly re-creates stressful situations. With this expanded awareness we are able to select a new, more open approach.

The Effortless Learning process presents an increasingly complex series of tasks. At some point in the process, your mind may be convinced that the task before you is impossible. If you make an attempt, however, you'll find that you *are* able to do it even though your mind will not understand how it happened. Then you will attempt something that appears to be even more difficult. You may try very hard, but you still won't be able to do it. Yet as soon as you stop trying, you will accomplish the task with ridiculous ease. Gradually you will become comfortable with a way of learning and being that has nothing to do with what you *think* you can do or how hard you are trying.

Effortless Learning is the ultimate step in the natural vision improvement process. It reopens the body/mind and anchors that new awareness—that new vision—in a new way of being in the world. As we expand, we spontaneously begin to live with more trust and less effort. We begin to rediscover the infinite potential that lies within. We can actually feel our pattern of narrow thinking expanding as our body/mind recalibrates itself.

How I Found My Effortless Genius on a Trampoline

After the initial phase of my vision improvement process, I began to reexamine my lifelong difficulty with reading. I could read, but it was so stressful that I avoided it whenever possible. I couldn't comprehend what I was reading no matter how many times I would read it over. I had struggled with this problem all through grade school, high school, college, and optometric school. Now I was a doctor with a reading difficulty—and a sense of inferiority. How could I be a real doctor if I had to struggle to read scientific journals? It seemed that the only way I could absorb new information was through direct experience.

When I shared this problem with some friends at an educational guidance center, they suggested that I come in and have an evaluation to assess my learning strengths and weaknesses—but I couldn't do that. I was afraid they would decide I wasn't smart enough to be a doctor, that I had gotten in through the back door. I was sure the test would confirm that I wasn't as smart as other people. After all those years, I was finally maintaining the illusion that I knew something, but if I took that test, they would discover the awful truth about me. So I turned down the offer.

For years I had been working with children who had visually related learning difficulties . . . a doctor with a learning disability treating children with learning disabilities. (It seems we are always drawn to heal ourselves in others.) I was finding the traditional concepts of "learning disability" and "attention deficit disorder" to be just as limiting and meaningless as the standard optometric procedures I had been taught in school. I kept thinking that there must be a better way of understanding and treating learning problems, and I felt that the answer must be related to the powerful links I was seeing between vision, movement, breathing, and thinking. What was the connection and how could it be put into practice?

I had heard about an Oregon optometrist, Dr. Robert Pepper, who was treating learning problems and improving athletic performance with trampoline exercises. His work was strongly recommended by a colleague, so I decided to go myself for a week of treatment. It turned out to be one of the most powerful turning points in my life, both personally and professionally.

Dr. Pepper took me through an extraordinary set of exercises, both on and off the trampoline. I started out standing on the floor. In the first exercise, he showed me a chart with a group of arrows pointing in different directions. He said, "Read across the rows and call out the direction of all the arrows." I could do that. I might make a few mistakes, but I could do that. At the end, he said, "Now call out the direction of the arrows and at the same time move both your hands in that direction." Okay. That wasn't so hard. Then he said, "Now do the same thing, but as you move your hands, make sure that your palms are also pointed in the same direction." It was only a little more complicated, but again, it wasn't so hard. So far, my mind could figure it all out.

Then he said, "Now call out the direction of the arrows and simultaneously move your hands in the opposite direction." I immediately choked up. My mind went into overtime and seemed to lock up. "Oh my God, oh my God," was all I could think. My hand went one way while my mind went the other way. "Should I say 'right'? Should I say 'left?'" My breath stopped. My vision blurred over. My body became as tense as a log. My head jutted forward, my back tightened up, and on the first arrow I loudly declared: "Reft!"

I recognized this reaction as the same feeling I had experienced in school. Whenever the teacher would ask me a question, my throat would get stuck, my mind and body would freeze, and my vision would blur. I suddenly realized that my internal dialogue was my own worst enemy. It had learned to interpret situations as stressful and then respond by creating so much anxiety that I couldn't function. To preserve my narrow thinking about myself, I had learned to ensure that I wouldn't succeed and to repeatedly create fresh proof of my own inadequacy.

Since I was regularly practicing Open Focus, I wondered why I couldn't stay in Open Focus while doing these exercises. I noticed that they required me to process a set of contradictory or nonlinear instructions. Since the conscious mind is limited in the number of activities it can process at once, I realized that my linear mind was overloading in the face of these multidimensional tasks. It would have to let go to allow the tasks to be done by some other level of my awareness.

As the session continued, I relaxed a bit and was able to accomplish increasingly complicated tasks while standing on the floor. Then I got on the trampoline. At first Dr. Pepper just asked me to jump and move my hands in little circles with each bounce. I didn't know that our hands automatically move in a circular pattern as we jump. I thought it was something extra that I had to remember to do.

Then he wrote a sentence on the board: "The train went by very fast." He said, "On every jump call out each letter in the sentence in sequence, and when you get to a space, just clap your hands." Well, it took me a couple of tries, but I got through that. Then he said, "Now every time you get to the letter 'T,' substitute a color instead." I did that. It wasn't that difficult. Then he said, "Now every time you get to a vowel, don't say anything." He just kept adding substitutions: "Every time you get to this, call out the name of a car, and every time you get to that, call out the name of an animal or a state," and so on. By the end, he had changed about thirty variables, but he had worked me up to it so gradually that I was eventually able to do it.

Just when I thought we were all done, he said, "Now turn around and do it without looking at the sentence." Again, I could only think, "Oh my God, oh my God." Then something magical happened. When I turned around, I began to see each letter in my mind's eye. I had always thought that visualization meant seeing the big picture all at once, but this wasn't like that at all. The letters came to me one at a time, exactly when I needed them. It was as if the Universe was saying, "If you're really trusting and patient, you'll get just what you need, just when you need it—not a second too soon or a second too late." I realized that that's the way life is meant to work. We get just what we need when we need it. The problem is that our mind wants to get it ahead of time so it can check everything out and feel in control.

As soon as I saw those images, I was able to let go and do the sentence in my mind's eye. Then Dr. Pepper said, "Now do the same thing . . . *backward.*" I couldn't do that! My mind panicked again. I thought that if I memorized the sentence, it would help, but I couldn't even *think* it backward. No matter how hard I tried, I was stuck; it seemed that I just couldn't get past this one. Finally my mind decided that this was hopeless and just gave up. As it let go, I suddenly saw the sequence in my mind's eye, just as I had earlier. Again, it was easy! I figured *this* had to be the end. So I turned around and said, "Okay, I did it."

Dr. Pepper responded, "No, no, stay turned around. Now do it backward again, but call out the first letter and then the last letter, the second letter and then the second to last letter, the third letter and then the third to last letter," and so on. This one really seemed to be impossible. Yet throughout the process, every time he upped the ante, I had learned something. I kept noticing how my mental anxiety was blocking my ability to move forward and that every time I started thinking, I held my breath. So somewhere during the task—I don't know how it happened—I just stopped thinking and started breathing, and it all became as smooth as silk. In fact, the task was so easy that I didn't even realize that I had done it successfully until Dr. Pepper started clapping. I just said, "Can I do it again?" After fluctuating in and out throughout the process, my vision was now crystal clear.

This was such a profound experience that when we were done, I threw myself onto the trampoline, laughing and crying at the same time. After all those years of self-doubt, I had finally found myself. I had so much more potential than I had ever dreamed. I knew that I couldn't do *this* and be stupid. The morning after I returned home, I walked into my friends' office at the guidance center and told them that I was ready to be tested. Later they told me my intelligence score was very high—and that was the end of my lifelong belief that I wasn't smart enough!

Years later, after seeing this wonderful process catalyze change for thousands of people, I realized that self-awareness is *the* key to self-transformation. It seems that our basic nature doesn't change that much. However, as we become more accepting of the person we've always been, our perception of ourselves expands dramatically. We learn to trust ourselves, we start to love and respect ourselves on a completely new level, and we become far more open and trusting in our everyday life.

I started adapting Dr. Pepper's work to my practice. He had been using it to improve competitive performance, but I had a different goal: to create an effortless mind/body state that would enhance learning and healing. So I revised his approach to enhance its power as a mirror of awareness. I wanted the process to develop spontaneously rather than exist as a set list of exercises. I began creating new exercises to fit the specific needs of each person I worked with. As you do the movement work yourself, remember it is a dynamic process that you never need to do the same way twice.

This was the origin of Effortless Learning, which leads you through a progressive series of paradoxical cognitive processes that *cannot be done with the mind.* You will learn that you can use memory, attention, rhythm, timing, visualization, gross and fine motor coordination—all at the same time—to accomplish something that you've never done before. But the only way to do this is to release your mental control.

Effortless Learning can be used to enhance learning and visual abilities in both adults and children. However, it's also been successful with those who are neurologically impaired, such as people with cerebral palsy or severe head trauma. Some of my clients had literally lost most of their memory as the result of head trauma, and were learning to rewire their mind/body connection.

In addition to the therapeutic value, these techniques enhance all levels of mind/body performance. I have used Effortless Learning techniques with members of the U.S. Olympic Team and world-class athletes. It has even helped world champions revive their stalled careers. These people all experienced profound change, but even more important, they all had *fun.* Effortless Learning is enjoyable, revealing, and dramatically enhances mind/body integration.

How can we do a problem-solving task without thinking? It's a paradox. It seems impossible. If you try to think your way through the exercises, you won't succeed. The only way to do them is without effort of any kind. You'll find yourself amazed as you disengage your mental control and begin to move beyond your previous limitations. As you do, your field will expand. All constricted areas of awareness, including vision, learning capacity, and attention span, will begin to open up. Your mind/body will become increasingly integrated. You'll learn to think and act by heart, even under stress.

Although I usually work with a trampoline or a rebounder (a very small, low trampoline), you don't need one for the Effortless Learning process. There are many powerful procedures you can do just standing on the floor. The next chapter presents a series of exercises to do while standing on the floor, and also describes the trampoline exercises. At home, you can use a small rebounder, which can be purchased in most department stores. (See Appendix A for ordering information.)

Once you become familiar with the basic idea, you can create your own exercises. They can be as complex or as simple as you like. If possible, work in pairs and have someone else guide you through the exercises; otherwise, you may not discover how far you can really go. Effortless Learning is also ideal as a family activity. The whole family can get involved and have fun at the same time.

16 How to Learn Without Effort

There is no way to know before experiencing.
—Dr. Robert Anthony

ALTHOUGH IT'S certainly helpful to work with a rebounder, you can get started on the Effortless Learning process at home without any special equipment. If at all possible, find a partner to give you the instructions, observe your process, and give you honest, supportive feedback. Before beginning, make sure that both you and your partner clearly understand the purpose and intention of the procedures. You can both read the following section and review it together.

One of the most important ingredients for healing or transformation is simply being present NOW. That's all that Effortless Learning is really about: It shows us how hard we must struggle when we *aren't* present and how effortlessly we succeed when we *are* present.

The purpose of the process is not to get the "right" answers. There are no "right" and "wrong" answers. The idea is simply to use the experiences that come up to notice and transform how you habitually respond to stressful situations.

What we usually call a "wrong" answer is simply a tangible reminder that we have somehow gotten out of the effortless flow. Instead of thinking, "Oh no, I messed up!" when you get that reminder, *thank it.* Then ask yourself, "What happened?" You don't need to analyze this question. You don't need to believe the mind's excuses—"I got confused," "I couldn't remember the instructions," "I couldn't see the chart." Simply notice what was happening to your awareness. Usually, after a "reminder" occurs, you realize that you actually started thinking, worrying, or anticipating a few seconds before it happened. Your partner may have noticed when you first started tensing up or holding your breath. What were you doing at that point? Where was your mind? Where was your awareness?

You may even notice that there is a particular place or symbol where you repeatedly get stuck. This symbol is your special friend, so make sure you thank it every time you get that feedback. If you still feel insecure because you've "made a mistake," ask yourself why. You aren't doing this to impress anyone else; you're doing it for you. Does the presence of your partner (who is probably a good friend, anyway) stimulate performance anxiety? Is this how you usually feel when you face a situation in which you feel you must "perform" for others?

Notice how fast you are going. We have been brainwashed to believe that faster is better: "The last one there is a rotten egg!" This simply adds more stress by taking us out of our comfortable internal rhythm. If you find yourself moving more quickly than is comfortable, get in touch with what is behind that. Did your schooling include the message "The faster the better"? Have you learned to speed up in response to feelings of stress in your work or daily life? How does that feel? Have your partner periodically remind you to give yourself permission to go at your own speed.

Finally, remember that Effortless Learning can only occur during open thinking. It is natural to experience some resistance as your analytical mind learns to let go of hard thinking, but as you allow yourself to breathe into your own rhythm and know that you are more than your linear mind, you will spontaneously enter a gentle, meditative state, similar to that of tai chi, yoga, or martial arts. Notice whatever is keeping you from that effortless flow. Is that resistance part of a pattern that you habitually experience? You don't need to do anything except notice it and allow it to be replaced by your spontaneous genius.

Part 1: Getting Started

The following is a very easy progression that allows you to proceed at your own pace. If you want to go very slowly, do just one additional step each day. Never move on to the next step until you can do the previous one effortlessly, without "reminders." At first, repeat the initial steps each time. After a week or so, you can start at a higher level.

If you are thinking of guiding another person through the Effortless Learning process, be sure to fully experience it yourself before you facilitate anyone else. Your experiential understanding extends only as far as the exercises you have mastered. This is especially important if you are working with a child, because you may need to proceed very slowly to avoid exceeding his or her level of proficiency.

You will need an arrow chart, which you can design yourself (see the following page). Take a piece of poster paper and draw on it five rows of five or six arrows each, randomly pointing in all four primary directions—left, right, up, and down. The arrows can be any width or length, as long as they are clearly distinguishable from one another. Hang the completed chart on a wall or place on an easel so that it is approximately at eye level and there is enough space in front of it for you to stand at varying distances as you do the procedures.

Remove your corrective lenses before you start. Begin by standing at a distance from which you can comfortably see the chart. If you're myopic, challenge yourself by taking one step away from the chart after you complete the first procedure. Proceed with the next exercise from there. Then take another step back to do the next procedure. How does that feel? If the chart appears blurry at first, don't give up just yet—you may be able to expand the boundaries of what you think you can see. Breathe, blink, feel your fear, and do the exercise anyway. Just notice what happens.

In a workshop, I was guiding a man I'll call Peter through the Effortless Learning process. Peter had worn a strong prescription for many years. I didn't check his acuity, but from looking at his

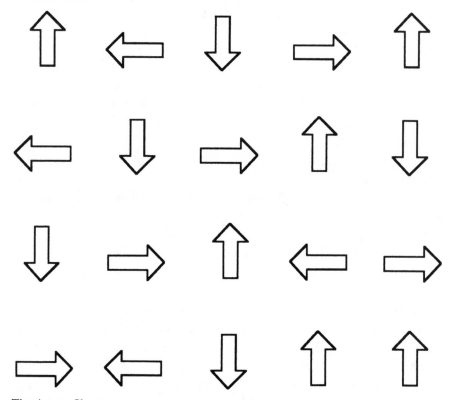

The Arrow Chart

glasses I'd guess it was around 20/300. I asked him to begin by removing his glasses and standing where he could comfortably see the chart. Peter moved up until he was five feet from the chart. He said that he could read the chart without stress at that distance, but I noticed that he was tense and was holding his breath tightly.

After each step of the process, I would ask him to step back a foot. Every time he moved back, we could see him thinking, "Uh-oh. My vision is too blurry. I can't see the chart this far away." At first he got even more tense, but then something interesting began to happen: He began to enjoy himself, and his mind started to let go. The group watched in amazement as he became more relaxed, spontaneous, and accurate with each step back.

By the time we finished fifteen minutes later, Peter had moved all the way to the opposite wall, about twenty-seven or twenty-eight feet from the chart. He was reading the chart accurately, having a lot of fun, and laughing heartily. So much for what we think we can't see!

If you're working alone, be sure to challenge yourself to move beyond your limitations. If the instructions sound as if they are within your comfort range, your linear mind won't have to let go. When you can work through the initial steps easily, continue adding more complex instructions until your mind says, "I can't do that!" That's the point at which your Effortless Learning process will really start.

In the beginning, you may have to continually remind yourself to breathe with each movement. However, this conscious direction will soon shift into an effortless, rhythmic flow, and each action will flow easily into the next without any breaks in your movement or awareness.

As you begin every step, notice how you may automatically start to *think about* or rehearse the instructions in your mind, but you don't need to prepare yourself—that actually just gets in your way. Listen to the instructions, take an easy breath, and begin.

Step One

After removing your glasses or contacts, find a comfortable distance from the chart. Stand in a relaxed position, with knees slightly bent, and become aware of your breathing.

Now move your head slowly and rhythmically in the direction that the first arrow is pointing and then back to center. Then move your head in the direction of the next arrow. Continue in this manner through every arrow in the chart—for example, if the first arrow is pointing right, move your head to the right; if the next arrow is pointing up, move your head up, and so on. Move rhythmically, very slowly, and take a breath between each arrow.

If you get to a "reminder" in which your head does not move in the direction of the arrow, stop and *thank that arrow*. What happened? How did your awareness stray out of the flow of the present? Then start over from the beginning.

After you finish, stop and ask yourself: Were your eyes moving in the direction in which your head was moving . . . or were they glued to the chart in front of you no matter which way your head moved? If you were keeping your eyes on the chart, try Step One again, but this time allow your eyes to move fully away from the chart each time your head turns away. Continue to breathe between each arrow and trust your spontaneous responses.

Step Two

Go through the chart again, but this time move your head in the *opposite direction* from each arrow—for example, if the first arrow is pointing right, move your head to the left. If the next arrow is pointing up, move your head down, and so on.

For this and all following steps, continue the procedure described in Step One—follow the chart rhythmically and meditatively until you reach the end of the chart, or a "reminder"—if you do, *thank that reminder.* How did you react when you noticed it? Where was your awareness just before that point? How long did it take you to notice that your awareness had strayed? Is the time between each "reminder" and your awareness of it getting shorter or longer? Usually, your awareness becomes sharper with practice. Each time, go back to the beginning of the chart until you can move through it effortlessly. *Always breathe easily and rhythmically between each arrow, and move very slowly.*

Step Three

This time keep your head still and simply move your eyes in the direction of each arrow.

By now, you are probably breathing comfortably between each arrow. So continue breathing and allow each movement of your eyes to naturally flow into the next movement, without returning to center.

Step Four

Again, keep your head still and move *only your eyes,* this time in the direction *opposite* each arrow. If the arrow is pointing left, move your eyes right. If the arrow is pointing up, move your eyes down. Continue to *breathe.*

Step Five

This time do not move your head *or* eyes. Simply call out the direction of each arrow while simultaneously moving your right hand in that direction. Make sure your palm is facing in the same direction your hand is moving.

Remember to *breathe* in between each arrow where you might otherwise be tempted to start thinking. As long as you keep breathing rhythmically, you'll remain in the effortless flow of the life force.

Step Six

Switch hands and do Step Five with the left arm. Again, make sure that the left palm is always facing in the direction the hand is moving.

Notice if you move more effortlessly in one direction than the other.

Step Seven

Call out the direction of each arrow while moving *both* hands in that direction. Again, make sure your palms are facing in the direction your hands are moving.

Step Eight

Call out the direction of each arrow and simultaneously move both hands in the *opposite* direction. Remember, move slowly.

If you find this instruction difficult, notice how stimulated your mind becomes—we believe that we must *think* in order to solve a difficult problem. But this kind of task can only be done *effortlessly.* Otherwise, it's like asking a pro football player to *think* about what he's doing while he's running for a touchdown. If he stops to consider what he's doing even for a second, he'll be tackled! So move slowly, keep breathing, and keep thanking your reminders.

Step Nine

Move both hands in the direction of each arrow and *call out* the opposite direction.

Let go of what you have just learned and do it the opposite way!

Step Ten

Now alternate steps eight and nine on each line: On the first row, call out the direction of each arrow and move your hands in the opposite direction. On the second row, move your hands in the direction of each arrow and call out the opposite direction. Continue to switch the instructions at the beginning of each line—and *breathe.*

Olympic Games

Step Eleven

For a real challenge, alternate Steps Eight and Nine *on each arrow:* On the first arrow, call out the direction of the arrow and move your hands in the opposite direction. On the next arrow, move your hands in the direction of the arrow and call out the opposite direction. On the third arrow, go back to the instruction for the first arrow. Continue in this manner, alternating the procedure for each arrow.

Remember to go much slower than your typical pace and to breathe rhythmically between each arrow.

Step Twelve . . . etc.

Make another arrow chart as before, but draw the arrows in different colors. Now start to alternate the instructions according to the color of the arrow—for example, on a red arrow you might call out the direction of the arrow and move your hands in the opposite direction. On a blue arrow you might move your hands in the direction of the arrow and call out the opposite direction, and so on.

You can use your imagination to come up with interesting additions, but here are a few suggestions.

Variation One

Follow the instructions for Step Eight *except* when you come to a blue arrow. Then call out your mother's name (or your father's name).

Variation Two

After you have mastered the first variation, make up another color substitution. It should be something different from the substitution for the first color. If the first color was the name of a person, the second color could be the name of a car or an animal, or an action, such as "Instead of speaking, clap your hands when you get to each red arrow."

Further Variations

Draw a chart with diagonal arrows—up right, up left, down right, and down left. Now go through the entire sequence from the beginning!

You might consider doing a series of these procedures every morning as a moving meditation. I have found that this practice has a wonderfully balancing and expanding effect on the system.

These procedures are just the beginning! The real fun starts when you get on the trampoline. As your feet leave the floor, your normal grounded sense of reality will shift, allowing a whole new level of awareness and learning to take place.

Part 2: Trampoline Games

It's important to begin the Effortless Learning process on your feet so that you become "grounded" in the basics before you jump into the air. On the ground, you will experience one level of awareness. When you leave the ground, something very different occurs.

We've seen that every time we think hard, we stop the breath and contract the body, but normally we are unaware of this—as long as our feet are on the ground! When we jump into the air, we open ourselves to a new perception of those habitual reactions. By thinking hard, we interrupt the spontaneous flow that keeps us in fluid motion. This manifests as a momentary loss of muscular control—our body may twist or contort, we may make funny faces—all because the mind is trying to *hold on*. We also seem to be more aware of all our feelings and sensations when our feet are off the ground.

So after doing the first series of procedures on the ground, you can move to the trampoline or rebounder. At first, simply practice jumping up and down while breathing and moving your hands in little circles with each jump: As you jump, allow your hands to move up and then spontaneously fall outward, in a circular motion.

These hand circles actually occur naturally as you relax your arms and hands, but at first many people will need to be shown how to do it: Throughout the circle, your fingers will remain together and your palms will remain down. Your hands will be at waist level and closest together when your feet hit the trampoline. If the exercise calls for you to do any clapping, you will clap at that point, but be sure your palms remain down and only turn toward each other during the clap. You will also do any other activities, such as calling out directions, as your feet hit the mat. The idea is: Feet hit, hands together, mouth speaks—simultaneously.

Once you are comfortable with the hand circles, try the following warm-up. Continue to breathe, circle your hands, and move effortlessly as you do it. If you have a partner, her role will be to help you notice whenever you begin to freeze up—whenever you hold your breath or stop moving your hands:

> Count by two's to twenty, counting one number on each jump. When that feels easy, begin to gradually add substitutions, one at a time. Proceed gradually and don't overload yourself. Add each substitution only after you feel comfortable doing the previous one.
>
> First, substitute the number 3 for the number 14. Next, substitute the name of a color for the number 4. Then, substitute a letter for the number 18, and then the name of an animal for the number 8.
>
> When you've done all that, do the whole process again, *backward.*

After warming up, you can begin any of the following "trampoline games." Each game moves from a simple to a more complex level of accomplishment, requiring a higher level of trust and awareness. The most challenging variations are the Olympic Games at the end of each procedure. You may not be able to do the Olympic variations until you have practiced the games for a while, so don't try to force yourself through them in the beginning. It's fine to do only the games that look interesting to you, but never move to the higher level of an exercise until you have successfully completed the basics—taking a shortcut just doesn't work. The Effortless Learning process is like building your dream house: You want to make sure every nail goes in straight!

Some of these games focus on a particular topic—working with numbers, letters, directions, and so on. If you are working with an area that has been difficult for you in the past, be patient with yourself, but don't avoid that subject just because you are thinking, "I'm not good at math," or "I always get my directions mixed up," or "I can't spell." Those beliefs actually show you where you can achieve the greatest breakthroughs in Effortless Learning!

For instance, the "Continuous Calculations" described below are a number exercise. Many people have a fear of numbers; they believe they "aren't good at math." But this technique is a completely different approach to working with numbers. It can actually help you heal your fear by showing that you can operate as effortlessly as a calculator. When you enter a formula into a calculator, the answer appears immediately. This technique works the same way. You stay fully present, and the answer simply comes through you. You have no idea where it comes from.

You may not believe you're "smart enough" to do math without thinking, but the greatest "human calculators" have extremely low IQs; they produce the result *without thinking.* They're called "idiot savants," and as Joseph Chilton Pierce explains in *Evolution's End: Claiming the Potential of Our Intelligence,*

> these people have an average IQ of 25. They are generally incapable of learning anything, few can read or write. Yet each has apparently unlimited access to a particular field of knowledge that we know they cannot have acquired . . . *[they] do not calculate, they simply respond to stimuli given,* if that stimuli is resonant with their narrow spectrum of ability.[1]

They can't even dial a phone number. But they can immediately tell you the answer to 17,991 times 46,521, or tell you the day of the week of a date tens of thousands of years in the past or future. And they do it, literally, as fast as a computer. How do they do it? They seem to be able to fully access one tiny fragment of the holographic field of intelligence. We, on the other hand, seem to have very limited access to the whole field. We know a little bit about a lot of things, while they know one tiny subject infinitely and effortlessly.

If there is a subject that you have had difficulty with that isn't covered in the exercises below, you can use it for your substitutions in the advanced versions of the techniques. For instance, if you feel that geography is an especially difficult subject, you can substitute the names of capitals, countries, or states whenever you get the chance.

I was working with a client I'll call Sheila. As we proceeded, we began to substitute the names of states for the letters in a sentence. I noticed that she was getting a little nervous, but I didn't know why. Finally, after substituting about three states, she broke down and told me, "Geography has always been my hardest subject. I just can't do this." She was almost crying.

By the end of the session, Sheila was able to recite almost all fifty states. How did that happen? She didn't suddenly memorize them; it was as if they had been hiding somewhere inside her awareness. We just found that door and opened it. That shift occurred spontaneously as she began breathing rather than *trying to think* about it.

For the trampoline games that use a chart of some kind, you can start by reading across the chart from left to right, as if you're reading a book. As you gain confidence, vary this by reading from right to left. The idea is to stay adaptable by doing things that you've never done before. So keep making up new ways to practice the games.

Jumping Arrows

The first technique is a continuation of the standing arrow exercises. The only difference is that now you'll be applying those same principles while jumping on the trampoline or rebounder. So we'll begin by going back to the basics:

Every time you jump, call out the direction of the next arrow—up, left, down, right. After you can do that effortlessly, call out the opposite direction—down, right, up, left. Make sure your hands are continually moving in little circles.

Then you can try a variation: Call out the direction of the arrow as if it were rotated a quarter turn clockwise—a down arrow becomes "left," a left arrow becomes "up," an up arrow becomes "right," and a right arrow becomes "down."

Just like in the earlier exercises, you will only be able do this by allowing the turn to enter your open awareness, not by analyzing it. Don't think about it, simply relax your focus and allow each arrow to appear to you. By not *doing* anything, you can access your effortless genius. Each time you do, you gain greater respect and trust in the spontaneous flow of your intelligence.

Next, you can rotate the arrow a quarter turn counterclockwise. Now the down arrow becomes "right," the right arrow becomes "up," the up arrow becomes "left," and the left arrow becomes "down."

Olympic Games

When you have effortlessly mastered both of these turns, you can alternate them: Rotate the first arrow a quarter turn clockwise and the next one a quarter turn counterclockwise. Keep switching between these two rotations on each arrow.

Jumping Color Arrows

This procedure uses a chart that consists of different colored arrows alternating with names of colors. The names of the colors are themselves drawn in various colors—the word "blue" on the first

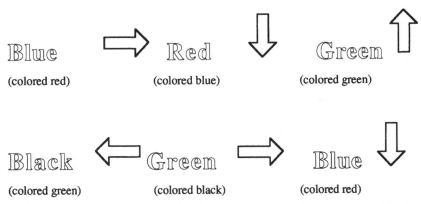

Colored Arrow Chart Instructions (Note: The arrows can be randomly filled in with any of the colors.)

row may be colored red, and "red" may be colored blue. "Green" may actually be colored green, and "black" may also be colored green. The next "green" may be black and the one after it may be red. After coloring in the words, draw the arrows in different colors as well.

Here's how to start using this chart: On each jump call out the name of the color and then the direction of the arrow. So this chart would read: "blue, right, red, down, green, up, black, left." After you can do that, call out the color *the word is written in and then the direction of the arrow:* red, right, blue, down, green, up, green, left. Then you can begin to alternate: direction, name of color, direction, color of word, direction, name of color, and so on.

Your imagination will be able to find many ways to use this chart, so continue to make up variations as you go along!

Mary Had a Little Lamb

For this one you need a simple sentence such as "Mary had a little lamb." On each jump call out one letter of the sentence, with a silent jump on the blank spaces: M-A-R-Y, silent jump, H-A-D, silent jump, and so on. After that, you can do the same thing again, except clap your hands on the blank spaces.

Next, read the sentence, clapping on the spaces, and count out a number every time you get to the letter "A." On the first "A," call out "one," and on the next "A," call out "two," then "three," and so on. Keep adding substitutions—maybe every time you get to the letter "E" you substitute a color. Next, every time you get to the letter "Y" substitute the name of a car. Then, every time you get to the letter "L" substitute the name of an animal. You can make up all kinds of substitutions, but be sure to add them slowly so that you master each addition before you move on.

First, do this reading the sentence forward; then do it reading backward. Then turn around and do it without looking at the chart.

Olympic Games

For the greatest challenge, alternate the letters from each end moving in toward the middle of the sentence, clapping on the spaces: "M, B, A, M, R, A, Y, L, clap, clap, H," and so on. When you can do that, add in your substitutions. Eventually you will be able to turn around on the trampoline and do any version without looking at the sentence. And when you do it without looking, your mind *really* lets go!

Continuous Calculation

This one is great for people who have a fear of math. First, write down two columns of five numbers between one and ten. We'll use this example:

4	8
7	5
1	2
6	9
3	10

Continuous Calculation Chart

You will be going *down* the column on the left and *up* the column on the right. On the first jump, call out the first number on the upper-left-hand corner: "four." Then take a silent jump and move to the number in the bottom-right-hand corner. This number is ten, but you don't call it out. Instead, on that bounce you call out the sum of four plus ten: "fourteen." Then you take another bounce and move to the second number in the upper-left column. You add that number to the sum and move to the second number in the lower-right column. You continue up and down the columns like this: "four," jump, "fourteen," jump, "twenty-one," jump, "thirty," jump, "thirty-one," jump, "thirty-three," jump . . . and so on.

Since you are doing all of this while jumping, there is *no time to compute it.* You simply open your awareness and allow the answers to come *through* you. The only thing holding you back is your fear, and as you relax and jump and breathe, your fear has nothing to hold on to. Once you can do this effortlessly, you can add more numbers. The columns can keep getting longer and longer.

Olympic Games

The game above just uses addition. The first Olympic variation alternates addition and subtraction. The first number is added to the second number, the next number is subtracted from that sum, the next number is added, the next number is subtracted, and so on. To do this, the linear mind has to get out of your way; you have to access your spontaneous intelligence.

If you'd like to go further, you can add multiplication and division. Remember: You're not calculating, you're simply allowing the answer to fall into place!

Jumping Formulas

Another type of math exercise uses formulas. For example, you might make up four formulas such as:

$$2 + 3 = \underline{\quad}$$
$$\underline{\quad} - 2 = 6$$
$$4 \times \underline{\quad} = 16$$
$$12 \div 3 = \underline{\quad}$$

Here you have formulas for addition, subtraction, multiplication, and division. On each jump call out each word of the equation in turn, including the number that is needed to fill in the next blank space: "two," "plus," "three," "equals," "five."

Olympic Games

When you can do that game easily, have your partner call out "plus one" or "minus one" (or any other single-digit number). You will add or subtract that number from the answer before calling it out. So if your partner calls out "minus four," your responses will be: "two," "plus," "three," "equals," "one."

Your partner can continue to call out a new number to add or subtract to each formula.

Fun with Balloons

This one is a great way for the whole family to have fun while enhancing mind/body integration: You won't need a trampoline, as it is usually done standing on the floor.

Fill up a large balloon and gather the family in a small circle, with one person holding the balloon. Select a simple word or sentence that all ages can spell, such as "Mary had a little lamb." (If you are doing it with children who can't spell yet, you can say the names of animals, colors, or parts of the body instead.)

The person who is holding the balloon calls out the first letter: "M!" and pushes it into the air, like a volleyball. As it comes down, the person who is closest to the balloon can hit it back, simultaneously calling out the next letter: "A!" Continue through the rest of the sentence, remaining silent when you hit the balloon on the spaces. It's most fun when everyone is able to participate. When a child gets a "reminder," help the child to figure out for him- or herself what happened—ask them questions rather than simply declaring, "That's wrong!" or "The answer was supposed to be ____!" Help them to reflect on their own process and understand for themselves.

Another creative approach is to start with just one word and keep adding words as you go along. The first person will call out a word, such as "Love." When that word and its space is spelled, the next person can call out any other word that would begin to form a sentence, such as "makes." And so on until the sentence is complete—perhaps "Love makes the world go round."

If you would like to learn more of these "family games," you might want to check out Dr. Ray Gottlieb's manual of paradoxical movement exercises for children (see Appendix A).

Olympic Games

As the family becomes more proficient, you can select increasingly difficult words or sentences, or add substitutions. Let the children take a turn in creating variations on the exercises. And remember that the most important element is to have fun!

Gold Medal Olympic Games— Paradoxical Eye Movements

Here's one of the most challenging games of all: When you get to the end of your session, lie down on the floor. Center yourself, breathe, and slowly begin to move your head to the right while moving your eyes to the left. Then switch and move your head left while moving your eyes right. This is a high-level neurological task, which will show you how effortless you have become. If you can do it in a relaxed flow, while breathing, you'll *know* that your mind-body integration has reached the Olympic level.

Switching Places

Once you have gone as far as you think you can go on the trampoline in one session, switch places with your partner. She gets on the trampoline, and you guide her. You can use your learning experience to create a series of games just for her.

You will soon discover that the guide has to be just as fully present and effortless as the other person. Otherwise, how will the guide know how the other person is doing? You have to do it along with her—*you* have to stay open while simultaneously observing *her* breathing and awareness. So whenever you work with another person you are also working with yourself. You are learning along with that person.

Doing the procedures on the trampoline is one level of awareness. Doing the procedures silently, while simultaneously observing another person doing them, requires a more complex level of awareness. But if you continue to breathe and stay open, you will be able to effortlessly guide the other person.

Always start wherever the person is comfortable, at a level she can succeed at with only a little effort. If in doubt, start off easy and let her build up to the harder procedures by showing both of you that she is ready. A child can start by just calling out directions or by silently moving his hand in the direction of the arrows. The substitutions can be names of animals or even the sounds that each animal makes. You can use any substitutions that are of interest to the person with whom you are working.

Allow each person to go at his or her own pace, but don't make it too easy, either. To expand our boundaries, we must reach a little farther each time. Every time we do something we've never done before, it stimulates our desire to reach farther. So give your partner a task that she is just able to do, and raise the ante a little bit each time. By gradually increasing the difficulty of the task, within an hour you might observe a person who was functioning at 20 percent of her learning potential go to 40 percent—permanently. The change has been permanently encoded in her system because she has learned it holographically and earned every step of the way.

You will notice yourself that once you've mastered a particular exercise, you'll be able to do it anytime, even if you haven't been "practicing" it. How are you doing it? Have you memorized it? No, it has nothing to do with memory or practice. You have simply encoded that procedure into your awareness. All you have to do to access it again is breathe and open your awareness.

In these games the body/mind learns to function with fluid spontaneity, like an Olympic athlete. There is a big difference between perfect technique and *mastery*. To be the best in the world, an athlete must transcend all of his technique and training. Technique can look very good, but mastery is spontaneous and *effortless*—because it comes from our holographic being, not from our mind.

17 Vision Quest

By Sonya Hagemann, O.D.
Calgary, Alberta, Canada

I BEGAN wearing glasses when I was twelve years old. I recall at that time being challenged with my body and relationships all changing at once. The hardest thing for me was being seen as a sexual being. Suddenly, men were treating me differently and since I didn't feel any different, I had no idea what to do. I remember deciding that if I didn't see it, I wouldn't have a problem anymore. I consciously chose not to see when someone was attracted to me. This was the beginning of a process I now call visual denial.

It was at that time I was found to need glasses. I remember crying for an hour when the optometrist told me this. I felt very over-whelmed and helpless at the prospect of spending my life behind glasses. More than worrying about looking ugly, I was grieving because I knew that a better way was available, but this doctor could not help me find it. I now know that moment of profound grief was actually the beginning of a search for my life's purpose.

Twenty years went by, with my prescription increasing steadily through the university years until it reached between −3.00 and −4.00 in each eye. My uncorrected vision was 20/400 in each eye. I wore my glasses constantly, never removing them even though I wanted to.

By the time I had been practicing optometry for four years, I had accomplished all my career goals and considered leaving the profession. I was bored and disillusioned with my work. I was developing a keen interest in body/mind medicine and human potential research and I needed to explore it more. When I went to work, I felt I had to repress that part of me in order to fit the image of a "good optometrist." I felt like a liar. I could tell there was a radical shift coming because I would oscillate between feeling very excited and very afraid. I felt afraid because I didn't know how the change would look, and yet the old way was draining the life out of me.

One day a light came on: If these body/mind theories were really true, then we all had the potential to heal anything within ourselves. If so, then I had the potential to see without glasses. I felt immense fear at the prospect, so I knew I was onto something. My vision needed to be improved if I was going to offer anything new to optometry. I had been asking for a vision for my life for so long. It occurred to me that the two questions were converging; they were one and the same question. I began a search for perfect eyesight and in the process found the vision of my life.

I met Jacob at a conference two months later. He suggested I remove my glasses just to see what would happen. Within minutes I felt really uncomfortable; although I could see him clearly, I felt very vulnerable. I went from anxiety to terror in minutes. The ground seemed to be falling away from me. I knew those feelings were the key to seeing clearly—if I could face them, I would see again.

I met many optometrists who were going through the same changes themselves, and their advice and support got me through the process of weaning myself from my glasses. I began to wear weaker glasses, never more than I needed at a given time. Every time I released more energy, I found I could reduce my prescription further. I did breathing exercises and yoga and started a regular meditation practice. I let myself express anything I needed to, whether it be having a breakdown at work or finally telling my father what I'd always wanted to. I quit my job just to take care of me for a while.

You know when you're living the right way when life becomes effortless. Everything you need comes to you without trying. I had a dream in which I could see clearly for a long distance. I felt ecstatic because I knew once it happened at the unconscious level, it would soon happen at the conscious level.

Shortly after that dream in November 1991, I attended Jacob's workshop and had the opportunity to work on the trampoline with him.

When he asked me to breathe, jump, and do an apparently impossible task of spelling a sentence backward and out of order, something incredible happened. Once I started, the letters just began to pop into my mind one at a time. This was an experience of nonthinking, of simply being rather than *trying* with my head. Logic and effort had always served me, but the beauty of that exercise is that those approaches do not work.

In that moment, I found the silence within myself—I call it Presence. Some call it God, Higher Self, a deep knowingness; the name doesn't matter. It was an opportunity to stop thinking and to allow myself to just have an experience. It is an experience of one's true self. I did not intellectually understand the task; I only knew I felt afraid to risk making a mistake. With Jacob's support I broke through the feat into a new level of being, and that's what seeing without glasses is all about.

The next morning I went to work without my glasses. Instead of putting them on when I felt stressed, I was forced to open up to Presence again because I'd left my glasses at home. When I did, I relaxed and found I could see again. I didn't have to think about how to do it; it just happened when I was willing, and I haven't really worn them since then.

It seems to me that the spirit is always the bottom line. When we can open up and trust ourselves, we can do anything. Medicine is now just beginning to recognize this interrelatedness of the body/mind/spirit. My search has been about bridging these aspects within myself. My single goal now is to help others wake up, see who they really are, and realize their own purpose. There was something incredibly powerful about one person seeing that I could do something, and when I was ready, his vision helped me change forever. It was in that moment I realized again we all have the power to help one another. Thank you, Jacob.

Epilogue: Open Living

Do not take life too seriously.
You will never get out of it alive.
—Elbert Hubbard

OPENING OUR awareness is an ongoing process. Every time we unfold one aspect of our lives, we begin to see possibilities for further expansion. An opening that may feel like the ultimate breakthrough at one point may later be seen as simply the prelude to the next miracle . . . and then the next, and on and on. Our potential for growth never reaches an end; even death may simply be a transition to a new level of development. No matter how far we evolve, as long as we are alive we will continue to experience expansion and contraction. Our goal is not some perfect state of permanent openness but the ability to flow through life's ins and outs as effortlessly as we can, learning from each experience we meet.

One morning in the fall of 1993 I awoke with a heavy heart; I was feeling a lot of shame. A few hours later I was standing at the kitchen sink, doing the dishes and gazing absentmindedly in front of me. It was a beautiful sunny day, but I felt heavy and dull. I wasn't thinking about how my feelings might be affecting my vision or my energy field. Then my eyes shifted up to look through the kitchen window, and in a flash my entire perceptive field opened up before my eyes. It seemed to be flooded with a brilliant light that exploded outward in all directions. It felt as if a star had erupted in front of me.

I realized in that moment that I had been "in the dark"—I had been seeing the world through a narrow gray tunnel. The tunnel had been invisible to me until the light appeared and the narrow opening expanded as if God was adjusting the focus of a very large camera lens. I could suddenly see just how much light I had been shutting out of my awareness. It felt like a miraculous gift.

This kind of instantaneous opening is very rare. I had experienced it when I discovered Open Focus while driving, twenty years before. But in 1973, I didn't see a gray tunnel; I just had a sense of expansion. I had no idea of the hole that I had been living in and looking through.

When the field contracts, we live in a gray tunnel all the time. And we can't imagine what it would be like to expand our awareness, because we have forgotten what openness feels like. So a sudden expansion can feel like a miracle, like a spontaneous freeing from our fear of life. Then we remember that miracles aren't rare but are everywhere around us.

Since we were raised to believe that vision improvement is impossible, this whole book has really been about creating miracles. And as we open our awareness to an expanded vision of our possibilities, we discover what we have always known: that miracles are the rule, not the exception; that spontaneous healing happens every day.

We all seem to be moving from the darkness of self-denial to the light of self-awareness. So how did we ever convince ourselves that effort and struggle are the essence of life rather than effortless joy and love? And how can we move into the light if we can't see the darkness? How can we reclaim our miraculous birthright?

The physicist David Bohm once said that all matter is frozen light.[1] Our receptivity to the light of life shapes our capacity to see, to know, and to feel. When we become frightened or contracted, we begin to see and feel selectively. We hold back the expression of our full potential for fear that our own power will overwhelm those careful limits. Vision problems are just one manifestation of our self-restriction. Clearing our vision is one way of saying "yes!" to more of life.

As our receptivity expands, we see the tremendous opportunities for growth and healing within all our challenges. We see how our lives seem to be programmed for continuous expansion. We see how miraculous life is meant to be. Open Focus is really about bringing ourselves back to our capacity for Open Living, which means allowing ourselves to freely express our full potential. It means releasing the struggle and fear that we have been trained to expect. It means accessing the spontaneous wisdom and vision of the heart. It means seeking our bliss and following it wherever it may lead us.

Goethe said that "light created the eye as an organ with which to appreciate itself." Rediscovering our true vision allows us to appreciate more of ourselves than we have ever dreamed possible. We are actually *human beamings*—holographic light sculptures. We are designed to be the *light of the world,* to continuously radiate our rainbow selves back to Creation.

Throughout the ages, saints and sages have taught that the core of Creation is an indescribable radiance of absolute love. Our minds cannot comprehend that luminous essence and our words cannot describe it. But we are designed to continuously reach toward that light by living as much of our potential as we can—and by seeing with the clarity and brilliance of our full awareness.

Appendix A
Vision Improvement Resources
(Products and Programs)

Beyond 20/20 Vision
Robert-Michael Kaplan, O.D.
RR 2, S26C39
Gibson, BC V0N 1V0
CANADA
604-885-7118
Fax: 604-885-0608

Cambridge Institute for Better Vision
Martin Sussman
65 Wenham Road
Topsfield, MA 01983
800-372-3937
508-887-3883

Information about Open Focus®:

Les Fehmi, Ph.D.
317 Mt. Lucas Road
Princeton, NJ 08540-2799
609-924-0782

For vision programs in Australia:

Janet Goodrich
Creative Vision Research
PO Box 999
Cabooltua, QLD
AUSTRALIA
71-985013

For vision improvement products, Ray Gottlieb's manual of exercises for children, and information about Jacob Liberman's lectures and workshops:

ULT
PO Box 520
Carbondale, CO 81623
800-81-LIGHT (800-815-4448)
303-927-0100
303-927-0101 fax

Appendix B
Behavioral Optometrists

If there isn't a behavioral optometrist near you (see pages 222 to 238), you can contact one of the organizations below for further referrals (they also offer books and educational materials on holistic vision care):

Optometric Extension Program Foundation
1921 E. Carnegie, Suite 3L
Santa Ana, CA 92705
714-250-8070

College of Optometrists in Vision Development
PO Box 285
353 H Street, Suite C
Chula Vista, CA 91910-0285
619-425-6191
619-425-0733 fax

IN THE U.S.A.

ARIZONA

Al Balthazor, O.D., F.C.O.V.D.
1013 N. Barkley
Mesa, AZ 85203
602-833-3433

Jefferson Hicks, O.D.
1127 Highway 43 South
Saraland, AZ 36571
205-675-2718

Richard Glonek, O.D., F.C.O.V.D.
10505 North 69th Street, 3-1000
Scottsdale, AZ 85253
602-483-0711

David Timochko, O.D.
1840 East Warner Road, Suite
   A103
Tempe, AZ 85284
602-820-9880

Robert Brooks, O.D.
8621 East 26th Place
Tucson, AZ 85710
800-977-0080

ARKANSAS

Lyman Squires, O.D., F.C.O.V.D.
PO Box 424
105 South Springfield Street
Berryville, AR 72616
501-423-2576

Jerry Shue, O.D.
324 West Pershing Boulevard
PO Box 2100
North Little Rock, AR 72115
501-753-3145

CALIFORNIA

Elliott Brainard, O.D.
Park Center for Health
4766 Park Granada, Suite 114
Calabasas, CA 91302
818-347-1910
   and
2562 State Street, Suite E
Carlsbad, CA 92008
619-434-5025

Peter Ross, O.D.
100 East Hamilton Avenue
Campbell, CA 95008
408-866-2020

E. M. Roberts, O.D.
374 East H Street, Suite 1708
Chula Vista, CA 91910
619-422-2020

Robert Wold, O.D.
353 H Street, Suite C
Chula Vista, CA 91910
619-420-3010

Wayne Nishio, O.D.
950 Herndon Avenue, Suite 101
Clovis, CA 93612
209-299-3179
   and
1726 Robertson Boulevard
Chowchilla, CA 93610
209-665-3797

Ami Patel, O.D.
2771 South Diamond Bar
   Boulevard
Diamond Bar, CA 91765
909-598-4393

Richard Stanley, O.D.
10305½ Lakewood Boulevard
Downey, CA 90241
310-862-5005

Kristy Remick, O.D.
River Rock Development
  Optometry Center
1004 River Rock Drive, Suite 131
Folsom, CA 95630
916-987-8086

Gary Scheffel, O.D., F.I.O.S.
1018 Riley Street
Folsom, CA 95630
916-983-9166

Gena Davis, O.D.
38820 South Highway 1, #107
Guacala, CA 95445
707-884-3937

Charles W. McQuarrie, O.D.
16152 Beach Boulevard, Suite
  250, East
Huntington Beach, CA 92647
714-841-4080

Robyn Rakov, O.D.
25301 Cabot Road, Suite 112
Laguna Hills, CA 92653
714-768-7225

Claude Valenti, O.D.
8950 Villa La Jolla Drive, #1114
La Jolla, CA 92037
619-453-0442

Carl Hillier, O.D.
7898 Broadway
Lemon Grove, CA 91945
619-464-7713

Melissa C. Hillier, O.D.
7898 Broadway
Lemon Grove, CA 91945
619-464-7713

Robert Sanet, O.D.
7898 Broadway
Lemon Grove, CA 91945
619-464-7713
  and
983 Lomas Santa Fe Drive,
  Suite C
Solana Beach, CA 92075
619-792-9060

William Henshaw, O.D.
801 South Fairmont
Lodi, CA 95240
209-334-2020

Sam Varon, O.D.
10771 Los Alamitos Boulevard
Los Alamitos, CA 90720
310-430-7515

Samuel Pesner, O.D.
133 Second Street
Los Altos, CA 94022
415-948-3700

Moses Albalas, O.D., O.M.D.,
  Ph.D.
12732 Washington Boulevard,
  Suite A
Los Angeles, CA 90066
310-306-3737

Alan Brodney, O.D.
10390 Santa Monica Boulevard,
  Suite 320
Los Angeles, CA 90025
310-553-7070

Richard Pozil, O.D.
10390 Santa Monica Boulevard,
  #320
Los Angeles, CA 90025
310-553-7070

Lawrence Simons, O.D.
9701 West Pico Boulevard,
   Suite 215
Los Angeles, CA 90035
310-284-8033

Herb Solomon, O.D.
1180 South La Brea Avenue
Los Angeles, CA 90019
213-933-9425

Steven Cohn, O.D.
833 Dover Drive, #9
Newport Beach, CA 92663
714-642-0292

Larry Jebrock, O.D.
1702 Novato Boulevard
Novato, CA 94947
415-897-9691

Iole Taddei, O.D.
1702 Novato Boulevard
Novato, CA 94947
415-897-9691

Jeffrey Anshel, O.D.
461 College Boulevard, Suite 1
Oceanside, CA 92057
619-758-0300
619-944-1200

Beth Gilman, O.D.
PO Box 3590
Quincy, CA 95971
916-283-2206

Steve Goedert, O.D.
1225 Eureka Way
Redding, CA 96001
916-221-9650
916-547-5345

Dale A. Fast, O.D.
1111 Howe Avenue, Suite 235
Sacramento, CA 95825
916-929-9162
916-447-5379

Marvin Schwartz, O.D., Ph.D.
3811 Florin Road, Suite 9
Sacramento, CA 95823
916-421-3311

Louis Katz, O.D., M.P.H., D.O.S.
4009 Governor Drive
San Diego, CA 92112
619-453-0444

Philip Smith, O.D.
3636 4th Avenue, Suite 200
San Diego, CA 92103
619-297-4331

Nina Getz, O.D.
Developmental Optometrist
121 South Del Mar Avenue,
   Suite A
San Gabriel, CA 91776
818-287-0401

Bradford G. Murray, O.D.
1556 Meridian Avenue
San Jose, CA 95125
408-445-2020

Burt Worrell, O.D.
1685 Westwood Drive
San Jose, CA 95125
408-267-2020

Kenneth A. Ethier, O.D.
845 Las Gallinas, #14
San Rafael, CA 94903
415-479-7305

Gerald Groff, O.D.
5290 Overpass Road, Suite 112
Santa Barbara, CA 93111
805-967-4693

Curtis Froid, O.D.
11 Dakota Avenue, Suite 4
Santa Cruz, CA 95060
408-423-5844

John Downing, O.D., Ph.D.
100 Santa Rosa Plaza
Santa Rosa, CA 95401
707-526-1881

George Ariyasu, O.D.
8783 Parthenia Place
Sepulveda (North Hills), CA
 91343
818-892-4017

Jim Mayer, O.D.
Mayer Eye Group
1337 East Thousand Oaks
 Boulevard, #110
Thousand Oaks, CA 91362
805-495-3937

Irving Werksman, O.D.,
 F.C.O.V.D.
Conejo Valley Optometry
 Center
372 North Moorpark Road
Thousand Oaks, CA 91360
805-495-0446

Stephen Chase, O.D.
22850 Crenshaw, Suite 104
Torrance, CA 90505
310-539-1210
714-895-3770

Dennis W. Hartman, O.D.
Turlock, CA 95380
209-667-6211

Craig Sultan, O.D.
3000 Alamo Drive, Suite 207
Vacaville, CA 95687
707-447-9899

Gary Etting, O.D.
7136 Haskell, #125
Van Nuys, CA 91406
818-997-7888

Donald Getz, O.D.
7136 Haskell Avenue
Van Nuys, CA 91406
818-997-7888
 and
2901 Wilshire Boulevard
Santa Monica, CA 90403

Clifford Fukushima, O.D.
5501 West Hillsdale Drive, #D
Visalia, CA 93291
209-625-5464

Phil Klingsheim, O.D., F.C.O.V.D.
11311 La Mirada Boulevard,
 Suite B
Whittier, CA 90604
310-946-3311

J. Richard Rishko, O.D.,
 F.C.O.V.D.
6319 De Soto Avenue, Suite 410
Woodland Hills, CA 91367
818-340-5796

COLORADO

Jay Highland, O.D., F.C.O.V.D.
PO Box 560
49 West Mill Street
Bayfield, CO 81122
303-884-9599

Tricia Brenner, O.D.
M. Stuart Tessler, O.D., F.C.S.O.
6979 South Holly Circle,
 Suite 105
Englewood, CO 80112
303-850-9499

Eva Strube, O.D.
1208 Washington Avenue
Golden, CO 80401-1145
303-279-3713

Cleve Armstrong, O.D., M.P.H.
801 South Public Road
Lafayette, CO 80026
303-665-3200

Marisa Atria, O.D.
255 Union Boulevard, #330
Lakewood, CO 80228
303-986-9554

Dorothy Parrott, O.D.
255 Union Boulevard, #330
Lakewood, CO 80228
303-986-9554

Roger Trudell, O.D.
800 South Hover Road, Suite 30
Longmont, CO 80501
303-651-6700

Marcy Rose, O.D.
7290 Samuel Drive, Suite 106
Westminster, CO 80221
303-428-7231

CONNECTICUT

Tyler Philpott, O.D.
5 School Street
Bethel, CT 06801
203-798-2020

Abraham Shapiro, O.D.
21 Polly Dan Road
Burlington, CT 06013
203-589-3593

Constantine Forkiotis, O.D.
437 Tunxis Hill Road, Box 741
Fairfield, CT 06430-0741
203-333-2772

Carl Gruning, O.D., F.A.A.O.,
   F.C.O.V.D.
33 Miller Street
Fairfield, CT 06430
203-255-4005

Susan Danberg, O.D.
212 New London Turnpike, #B-2
Glastonbury, CT 06033
203-657-9189

Jerrold E. Blum, O.D.
282 Railroad Avenue
Greenwich, CT 06830
203-625-0541

Ira Schwartz, O.D.
420 Long Hill Road
Groton, CT 06340
203-445-4277

Rhonda Greifinger, O.D.
40 Melon Patch Lane
Monroe, CT 06468
203-261-3422

Mark Feder, O.D.
5 Eversley Avenue
Norwalk, CT 06851
203-853-1010

Randy Schulman, O.D.
5 Eversley Avenue
Norwalk, CT 06851
203-853-1010

Alphonse Inclima, O.D.
415 Main Street
West Haven, CT 03713-6516
203-934-5126

Kenneth L. Burke, O.D.
175 Main Street South
Woodbury, CT 06798
203-263-3391

FLORIDA

William Clement, O.D.
PO Box 1099
123 West Oak Street
Arcadia, FL 33821
813-494-2662

Lawrence D. Lampert, O.D.
7035 Beracusa Way, #101A
Boca Raton, FL 33433
407-391-3334

Rick Morris, O.D.
19635 Street Road 7, #50
Boca Raton, FL 33498
407-451-0524
407-451-3916

Daniel Fleming, O.D.
2305 Oleander Avenue, #1
Fort Pierce, FL 34982
407-465-6616

Sheldon Kreda, O.D.
5450 North University Drive
Lauderhill, FL 33351
305-749-0000

Albert Sutton, M.S., O.D.
820 Lake View Drive
Miami Beach, FL 33140
305-861-8415
305-865-6783 fax

Ralph Mead, O.D.
1225 East Mount Vernon
Orlando, FL 32803-5466
407-896-4511

Walter Chao, O.D.
7867 Pines Boulevard
Pembroke Pines, FL 33024
305-966-4335

Michael Phillips, O.D.
5100 Central Avenue
St. Petersburg, FL 33707
813-321-1101
813-327-5302

John Walesby, O.D.
2802 West Waters Avenue
Tampa, FL 33614
813-915-0755

Stephen C. Franzblau, O.D.
6802 Forrest Hill Boulevard
West Palm Beach, FL 33413
407-439-2020

GEORGIA

Sharon Berger, O.D.
1190 Grimes Bridge Road
Roswell, GA 30075
404-992-7620

Daniel Gottlieb, O.D.
Gottlieb Vision Group
5462 Memorial Drive, Suite 101
Stone Mountain, GA 30083
800-666-7484
404-296-6000

HAWAII

Glen Swartwout, O.D.
311 Kalanianaole Avenue
Hilo, HI 96720
808-934-3235
800-788-2442

Clayton Gushiken, O.D.
2353 South Beretania Street,
   Suite 101
Honolulu, HI 96826-1413
808-941-3811

Barbara J. Dirks, O.D., M.Ed.
80 Mahalani Street
Wailuku, HI 96793
808-243-6234

IDAHO

Jeffrey Johnson, O.D.
Family Vision Clinic
501 North Curtis Road, Suite A
Boise, ID 83706
208-377-1310

Kenneth Cameron, O.D.
PO Box 1487
421 Church Street
Sandpoint, ID 83864
208-263-9589

and

226 West Main Street
Hope, ID 83836
208-264-5000

ILLINOIS

Harry Sirota, O.D.
5052 North Sheridan Road
Chicago, IL 60640
312-561-8918

Jeffrey Getzell, O.D., F.C.O.V.D.
1822 North Ridge
Evanston, IL 60201
708-658-4370
708-866-9850

and

19 North Main Street
Algonquin, IL 60102

Michael Zost, O.D.
1434 Waukegan Road
Glenview, IL 60025
708-657-8787

Dominick Maino, O.D.
4970 North Harlem Avenue
Harwood Heights, IL 60656
312-777-7838

Irving Peiser, O.D.
7851 West Ogden Avenue
Lyons, IL 60534
708-447-1515

Deborah Gail Zelinsky, O.D.,
    F.C.O.V.D.
244 Lagoon Drive
Northfield, IL 60093
708-501-2020

James Blumenthal, O.D.
104 West 144th
Riverdale, IL 60627
708-849-4040

Albert Freedman, O.D.,
    F.C.O.V.D.
Vision Development
3600 East State Street
Rockford, IL 61108
815-398-9393

Sharon Luckhardt, O.D.
136 North Cass
Westmont, IL 60559
708-969-2807

INDIANA

James Wessar, O.D.
525 West 38th Street
Anderson, IN 46013
317-649-2278

Merrill Allen, O.D., Ph.D.
Indiana University School of
    Optometry
800 East Atwater Street
Bloomington, IN 47405
812-855-7663

IOWA

Donald Hansen, O.D.
1923 Main Street
Davenport, IA 52803
319-324-3241
319-355-4684

David N. Hansen, O.D.
2600 Grand Avenue
Des Moines, IA 50312
515-243-1667
515-225-0366

KANSAS

Lowell Goodwin, O.D., F.C.O.V.D.
704 North Main Street
Garden City, KS 67846
316-276-2261

Jaryl Ollenburger, O.D.
359 North Highway 81
PO Box 696
Hesston, KS 67062
316-327-2800

Louis Mogel, O.D.
1001 North Main
Hutchinson, KS 67501
316-663-5417

Tony Powers, O.D.
6 East 2nd Street
Hutchinson, KS 67501
316-663-6060

A. L. Young, O.D.
1001 North Main
Hutchinson, KS 67501
316-663-5417

Norbert Stigge, O.D.
1202 Moro
Manhattan, KS 66502
913-539-6051

Verne Claussen, O.D.
631 Lincoln, Box 27
Wamego, KS 66547
913-456-2236

MAINE

Bradford Smith, O.D.
15 Western Avenue
Augusta, ME 04330
207-623-2020

Edward Godnig, O.D.
46 Dow Highway
Eliot, ME 03903
207-439-2164

Larry Ritter, O.D., M.S.
151 Main Street
Westbrook, ME 04098
207-854-1802

MARYLAND

Stanley A. Applebaum, O.D.
6509 Democracy Boulevard
Bethesda, MD 20817
301-897-8484

Marsha Kotlicky, O.D.
Michael Kotlicky, O.D.
308 South Main Street
Mount Airy, MD 21771
301-829-1910

MASSACHUSETTS

Michael Smookler, O.D.
Eye Care of South Brookline
1004A West Roxbury Parkway
Brookline, MA 02167
617-469-0015

Cathy Stern, O.D., F.C.O.V.D.,
   F.C.S.O.
27 Harvard Street
Brookline, MA 02146
617-277-7754

Antonia Orfield, O.D.
29 Inman Street
Cambridge, MA 02139
617-868-8742
   and
New England Eye Institute
1255 Boylston Street
Boston, MA 02215
617-262-2020

Harvey Schneider, O.D.
336 Baker Avenue
Concord, MA 01742
508-369-4453

Wilbert Libbey, O.D.
66 Eastern Avenue
Dedham, MA 02026
617-326-1256

Earl Lizotte, O.D.
PO Box 711
176 Main Street
Easthampton, MA 01027
413-527-4881

Solomon Slobins, O.D.
1200 Robeson Street
Fall River, MA 02720-5508
508-673-1251

Theresa J. Ruggiero, O.D.
139A Damon Road
Northampton, MA 01060
413-586-5002

MICHIGAN

Louis W. Schueneman, O.D.
1415 Center Avenue
Bay City, MI 48708
517-893-7565

MINNESOTA

Robert Zwicky, O.D.
2550 University Avenue West,
   Court International Building,
   Suite 163 South
St. Paul, MN 55114
612-645-8124

MISSISSIPPI

Roderick Fields, O.D.
Vision Therapy Center of South
   Mississippi
240 Eisenhower Drive, Bldg. H
Biloxi, MS 39531
601-388-6161

MISSOURI

David Coleman, O.D.
Coleman Family Eyecare Center
1651 West 7th, #1
Joplin, MO 64802
417-782-3488

David Luke, O.D.
113 East Promenade
Mexico, MO 65265
314-581-3824

NEBRASKA

Kerri Dietz Pillen, O.D.
1810 Wilshire Drive
Bellevue, NE 68005-3680
402-291-6133

NEVADA

Richard Meier, O.D., F.C.O.V.D.
3201 Lakeside Drive
Reno, NV 89509
702-825-0559
702-825-3939 fax

NEW JERSEY

William Moskowitz, O.D.,
F.C.O.V.D., F.A.A.O.
245 Union Avenue, Suite 2C
Bridgewater, NJ 08807
908-725-1772

Leonard J. Press, O.D.
Family Eyecare Associates
15-01 Broadway, Suite 9
Fair Lawn, NJ 07410
201-794-7977

Errol Rummel, O.D., F.C.O.V.D.,
F.A.A.O.
Adult & Pediatric Eyecare
2206 West County Line Road
Jackson, NJ 08527
908-364-4111

Roy Soloff, O.D.
1401 New Road
Linwood, NJ 08221
609-653-1800

Stuart M. Rothman, O.D.
25 West Northfield Road
Livingston, NJ 07039
201-992-0998

Stanley Levine, O.D., F.C.O.V.D.
240 Amboy Avenue
Metuchen, NJ 08840
908-548-3636

Jeffrey Zlotnick, O.D.
39 Bridge Street
Metuchen, NJ 08840
908-549-3555

NEW MEXICO

Steven M. Glover, O.D.
509 West Alameda
Roswell, NM 88201
505-622-5371

Sam Berne, O.D.
1300 Luisa Street, Suite 4
Santa Fe, NM 87505
505-984-2030

NEW YORK

Wendy Josephs, O.D.
420 12th Street, E2R
Brooklyn, NY 11215
718-788-4278
and
1036 Third Avenue
New York, NY 10021
212-447-7816

Thomas Steinmetz, O.D.
1320 52nd Street
Brooklyn, NY 11219
718-435-0220
and
401 Broadway
Lawrence, NY 11559
516-374-3320

Gerald Wintrob, O.D.
380 Marlborough Road
Brooklyn, NY 11226
718-856-2020

Richard O'Connor, O.D.
411 Main Street
East Aurora, NY 14052
716-652-0870

Gary Weiner, O.D.
175 Main Street
Fishkill, NY 12524
914-896-6700

Larry Wallace, O.D.
322 North Aurora Street
Ithaca, NY 14850
607-277-4749
607-272-1833

J. Baxter Swartwout, O.D.
400 Troy-Schenectady Road
Latham, NY 12110
518-785-7891

Harvey Estren, O.D.
164 North Wellwood Avenue
Lindenhurst, NY 11757
516-226-2313

Robert Byne, O.D.
Medical Arts Center
572 Route 6
Mahopac, NY 10541
914-628-3750

Martin Birnbaum, O.D.
515 Herricks Road
New Hyde Park, NY 11040
516-741-3332

Joseph Shapiro, O.D.
Center for Unlimited Vision
80 Fifth Avenue, Suite 1105
New York, NY 10011
212-255-2240

Ray Gottlieb, O.D.
336 Berkeley Street
Rochester, NY 14607-3311
716-461-3716

Marc Grossman, O.D.
20 Chestnut Street
Rye, NY 10580
914-967-1740
    and
3 Paradise Lane
New Paltz, NY 12561
914-255-3728

Albert Tyroler, O.D.
71 Barker Drive
Stony Brook, NY 11790
516-751-3781

    and
54 Terry Street
Patchogue, NY 11772
516-475-2025

NORTH CAROLINA

Cathy Doty, O.D.
New Bern Family Eye Care
1200 Simmons Street
New Bern, NC 28560
919-633-0016

OHIO

Paul Newman, O.D.
279 South Main Street
Akron, OH 44308
216-253-1627
216-836-4628

Brenda Heinke Montecalvo, O.D.
1546 Marsetta Drive
Beavercreek, OH 45432
513-429-2332

David Muth, O.D.
1125 Congress
Cincinatti, OH 45246
513-821-3296

Heath Gilbert, O.D.
813 Troy Street
Dayton, OH 45404
513-228-2020

Richard Horn, O.D.
6580 North Main Street
Dayton, OH 45415
513-275-3056

Carole Burns, O.D., Mark Wright,
    O.D., Kyla Cologgi, O.D.
185 South State Street
Westerville, OH 43081
614-898-9989

OREGON

Dr. Sandra Landis
14385 Southwest Allen
   Boulevard, Suite 102
Beaverton, OR 97005
503-646-8592

Garry Kappel, O.D.
17221 Southeast Oatfield Road
Milwaukie, OR 97267
503-653-2323
503-653-9872 fax

Bruce Wojciechowski, O.D.,
   I.C.O.V.D.
7831 Southeast Lake Road
Milwaukie, OR 97267
503-652-1771

PENNSYLVANIA

Elmer Ebeck, O.D.
101 Smith Drive, Suite 111
Cranberry Twp, PA 16066
412-776-5888

Christa Roser, O.D.
2791 South Queen Street
Dallastown, PA 17313
717-741-5531

Joseph Bytof, O.D.
7 North Baltimore Street
Dillsburg, PA 17019
717-432-4911

Robin Sapossnek, O.D.
930 Henrietta Avenue
Huntingdon Valley, PA 19006
215-663-5933

Arnold Bierman, O.D.
PO Box 1369
2302 North Broad Street
Lansdale, PA 19446-0749
215-822-1365

Elisa Haransky-Beck, O.D.
106 Trotwood Drive
Monroeville, PA 15146-4355
412-372-3016

Ellis Edelman, O.D.
313 North Newtown Street
   Road, Box 107
Newtown Square, PA 19073
610-356-1889

Steve Gallop, O.D.
313 North Newtown Street Road
Newtown Square, PA 19073
610-356-7425

Jacob Parker, O.D., Ph.D.
8595 Bustleton Avenue
Philadelphia, PA 19152
215-722-1133
215-728-7513

Arthur Seiderman, O.D., M.A.,
   F.C.O.V.D., F.A.A.O.
Plymouth Valley Professional
   Center
919 East Germantown Pike,
   Suite 4
Plymouth Meeting, PA 19401
610-279-8900
215-885-8900

Stanley Hozempa, O.D.
215 Ferguson Avenue
Shavertown, PA 18708
717-675-5072
717-675-5116

Charles Steinberg, O.D.
430 East Oakview Drive
Waynesburg, PA 15370
412-852-2276

PUERTO RICO

Drs. Pico, Tort & Gorbea
Optometras Pico Tort y Gorbea
Calle 2 #J-12-A, Ext. Hnas Davila
Bayamon, PR 00959
809-780-0677

RHODE ISLAND

Edward Lyons, O.D.
989 Reservoir Avenue
Cranston, RI 02910
401-943-1122

SOUTH CAROLINA

John Brinkley, O.D.
426 Bush River Road
Columbia, SC 29210
803-798-8111

Mark Dean, O.D.
Grand Strand Vision Service
4405 Socastee Boulevard,
   Suite J
Myrtle Beach, SC 29575-8764
803-293-1555

Alva Pack, O.D.
399 East Henry Street
Spartanburg, SC 29302
803-585-0208

TENNESSEE

James Miller, O.D.
628 East 10th Street
Cookeville, TN 38501
615-526-2143

TEXAS

Teresa Peck, O.D.
1713 East Highway 35
Angleton, TX 77515
409-849-7321

O. Reynolds Young, O.D.,
   F.C.O.V.D., F.A.A.O.
6036 Sherry Lane
Dallas, TX 75225
214-361-1300
214-361-7310 fax

Dhavid Cooper, O.D.
2055 Westheimer, Suite 115
Houston, TX 77098
713-520-6600
713-522-7905

Catherine West, O.D.
14741 Pebble Bend, Suite B
Houston, TX 77068
713-440-3286

John Juengerman, O.D.,
   F.C.O.V.D.
556 Bedford-Euless Road
Hurst, TX 76053-3924
817-268-2010

David Saul Mora, O.D., Ph.D.
1601 Corpus Christi
Laredo, TX 78043
210-726-1007
210-724-4009

VIRGINIA

Dennis Cantrell, O.D.
7611 Little River Turnpike,
   #303W
Annandale, VA 22003
703-941-3937
703-437-6406

Alan L. Sikes, O.D.
Burke Professional Center
9002 Fern Park Drive
Burke, VA 22015
703-978-5010
703-569-3757

A. Gregory, O.D., and Alan Toler,
O.D.
3026 West Cary Street
Richmond, VA 23221
804-359-6646

and

1407 Westover Hills Boulevard
Richmond, VA 23225
804-231-9151

Sidney Slavin, O.D.
4883 Finlay Street
Richmond, VA 23231
804-222-3653
804-741-2085

Robert Titcomb, O.D.
Haygood Medical Center
1020 Independence Boulevard,
#307
Virginia Beach, VA 23455
804-460-3688

WASHINGTON

Mark Robertson, O.D.
PO Box 309
Chelan, WA 98816
509-682-4021
509-682-3492

Curtis R. Baxstrom, O.D.
NW Vision Development Center
33919 9th Avenue South,
Suite 101B
Federal Way, WA 98003
206-661-6005
206-925-5221

E. Lynn Burge, O.D.
Harborview Vision Clinic
7244-700 West
Oak Harbor, WA 98277
206-675-2295

and

Harborview Vision Clinic
Kens Korner
Clinton, WA 98236
206-341-6959

William Nielsen, O.D.
PO Box 85147
Seattle, WA 98177
206-362-6624

WISCONSIN

Randall Melchert, O.D.
12750 West Capitol Drive
Brookfield, WI 53005
414-781-2020

Garth Christenson, O.D.
706 19th Street, Suite 4
Hudson, WI 54016
715-381-1234

Richard Foss, O.D.
2303 State Road
LaCrosse, WI 54601
608-788-4300

Paul Johnson, O.D.
146 North Brown Street
Rhinelander, WI 54501
715-362-2788

WYOMING

Sue Lowe, O.D.
Snowy Range Vision Center
301 South 8th Street
Laramie, WY 82070
307-742-2020

INTERNATIONAL

AUSTRALIA

Peter Fairbanks, O.D.
45 Lydiard Street South
Ballarat, VIC 3350
AUSTRALIA
05-3031-2122

Stephen Leslie, O.D.
Dannell & Gollop
Carousel Centre, Albany
   Highway
Cannington, WA 6107
AUSTRALIA
61-9-451-8722
61-9-387-6604

Anthony Hogan, O.D.
PO Box 697
Casino, NSW 2470
AUSTRALIA
06-662-1655
06-662-3983

Peter Woolf, O.D.
Hamilton, NSW 2302
AUSTRALIA
01-847-6420

A. S. Tan
Shop 12, Quakers Court
Quakers Road
Quakers Hill, NSW 2763
AUSTRALIA
02-626-3880
   and
8 Henley Road
Home Bush West
NSW 2140
AUSTRALIA
02-746-6016

Simon Grbevski, O.D.
Stephen J. Daly, O.D.
458 Princes Highway, Rockdale
Sydney, NSW 2216
AUSTRALIA
02-597-3030
02-597-6413 fax

BELGIUM

Naegels Guy, O.D., F.C.O.V.D.
Bacchuslaan 19
2600 Antwerpen
BELGIUM
03-235-6710

CANADA

Sonja Hagemann, O.D.
1990 Kensington Road NW
Calgary, ALB T2N 3R5
CANADA
403-270-4100
403-286-5135
   and
1910 Bowness Road Northwest
Calgary, ALB T2N 3K6
CANADA
403-283-2996 fax

Robert-Michael Kaplan, O.D.,
   M.Ed.
Beyond 20/20 Vision
RR#2, Site 26, Comp. 39
Gibsons, BC V0N 1V0
CANADA
604-885-7118
604-885-0608 fax

Viktor Kuraitis, O.D.
282 Linwell Road, #203
St. Catharines, ONT L2N 6N5
CANADA
905-935-1440

DENMARK

Steen Saust, O.D.
Hans Taersbol, O.D.
Buus Optik
Algade 40
4000 Roskilde
DENMARK
45-42-35-40-14

FRANCE

Christian Mona, Optometriste
Lyne Salama, Optometriste
13 Rue de la Viguerie B.P. 47
47800 Miramont de Guyenne
FRANCE
53-93 81 78

INDIA

Goutam Mukherjee, O.D.
Arambagh, Hooghly 712601
INDIA

ITALY

Domenico Intelisano, O.D.
via Pentapoli 73
96010 Priolo (SR)
ITALY
0931-767908
0931-767503

Gianni Greco, Optometrist
via Mariani 22 48100
Ravenna
ITALY
011-39-544-39232

Marino Formenti, O.D.
via Brenta Vecchia, 47
30171 Venezia-Mestre
ITALY
041-940094
0336-457730

NETHERLANDS

Robert Werrelman, O.D.
150 Kruisstraat
5612 Cm Eindhoven
NETHERLANDS
040-437619

Will Kock, O.D.
Herenstraat 31
1211 BZ Hilversum
NETHERLANDS
035-233541

Jan W. Dijkhof, O.D.
Dijk 46
1811 Mc Alkmaar
NETHERLANDS
072-117235
022-091893

NEW ZEALAND

Adrian Young, Dip. Opt.
Box 13863
Onehunga, Auckland
NEW ZEALAND
649-6369321
649-5245637 (home)

NORWAY

Jon Thoresen, O.D.
Stortorvet 5/7 Pb. 313
7601 Fredrikstad
NORWAY
69-31 15 38
69-31 62 25 fax

PHILLIPINES

Gloria Y Husted, O.D.
Medalle Bldg, R302-B, Osmena
    Boulevard
Cebu City
PHILLIPINES

SOUTH AFRICA

John Carey, O.D.
DOCARE
4th Floor, 20 Monument Street
Krugersdorp, 1740
SOUTH AFRICA
011-953 1856
011-472 1096

SPAIN

Jose Maria Argaluza, O.D.
Av. Basagoiti Etb., 55 (Optica)
48990 Algorta, Getxo-Bizkaia
SPAIN
94-491-05-47
94-491-00-69 fax

Appendix C
Natural Vision Improvement Practitioners

IN THE U.S.A.

ARIZONA

L. Marc Haberman, B.A., L.M.T.
Natural Balance Health Service
3150 East Presidio Road
Tucson, AZ 85716
602-881-4582

CALIFORNIA

Sean P. Mullen
Vision Improvement Center
PO Box 574
Berkeley, CA 94701
510-215-2020

Patricia Cavanagh
PO Box 1744
Campbell, CA 95009
408-249-4898

Denise Hornbeak, NVIP, EC, CLP
2317 Oxford Avenue
Cardiff, CA 92007
619-634-2325

Jerriann J. Taber, Ph. D.
Vision Training Institute
11303 Meadow View Road
El Cajon, CA 92020
619-440-5224
619-565-2020

RiAnn Healy
PO Box 477
Forestville, CA 95436
707-996-4368

Lisa Biskup
7781 North Baird
Fresno, CA 93720-0238
209-299-9433

Dr. John M. Hanson
Brain Development Center
5328 West 142nd Place
Hawthorne, CA 90250
310-643-9882

Richard Oliver, Jr.
13661 Acorn Patch Lane,
    Suite 100
Poway, CA 92064
619-689-6151

Janine Lee Riggle
Excellent Eyesight
629 Avenue A
Redondo Beach, CA 90277
310-316-3780

Verlin Burris
Vital Eyes
2291 Hurley Way
Sacramento, CA 95825
916-929-0180

Parents Active for Vision
    Education
9620 Chesapeake Drive, #105
San Diego, CA 92123
619-467-9620, 800-PAVE-98
619-467-9624 fax

Carrie Anderson
PO Box 470393
San Francisco, CA 94147
415-441-8683

Thomas R. Quackenbush
Natural Vision Center of San
    Francisco
PO Box 16403
San Francisco, CA 94116-0403
415-665-2010

Lee Hartley, Ed.D.
4020 Moorpark Avenue, #117
San Jose, CA 95117
408-249-6943

Patti Lawrence White
Motion Quest Associates
731 South Highway 101, Suite 2E
Solana Beach, CA 92075
619-792-5483

Margaret L. Yeomans
N'Tellect Center
990 Highland Drive, Suite 102
Solana Beach, CA 92075
619-689-6151

Lisette Scholl
PO Box 540
Templeton, CA 93465
805-434-1352

Nancy Papagni
5399 Annapolic Court
Ventura, CA 93003
805-650-9855

COLORADO

June Kirkwood, R.N., B.S.N.
318 Oak Lane
Aspen, CO 81611
303-925-4865

Deborah Banker, M.D.
1905 9th Street
Boulder, CO 80302
303-754-7858

Janet Herbst, M.S.Ed.
1208 Washington Avenue
Golden, CO 80401-1145
303-279-3713

HAWAII

Karen Peterson, M.A.
#109 PO Box 356
Paia, Maui, HI 96779
808-573-3109

ILLINOIS

Ron Deyo, D.C.
Deyo Chiropractic Center
Route A8 South
PO Box 147
Mount Carroll, IL 61053
815-244-2091

KENTUCKY

Pauline Johnson
7133 Johnson Road
London, KY 40741
606-878-1907

MAINE

Rosemary Gaddum Gordon,
   D.B.O., M.A.
Lightwater
17 Mast Cove Road
Eliot, ME 03903
207-439-8522

MASSACHUSETTS

Trudy Eyges
37 Day School Lane
Belmont, MA 02178
617-484-6833

Rosemary Gaddum Gordon,
   D.B.O., M.A.
Cambridge Health Associates
335 Broadway
Cambridge, MA 02139
617-354-8360

MINNESOTA

Kathy DeBoer
A Chance to Grow
3820 Emerson Avenue North
Minneapolis, MN 55412
612-521-2266

NEW YORK

Frank Nochimson, M.D.
416 74th Street
Brooklyn, NY 11209
718-833-5197

Leonie Newman
315 East 72nd Street, #1D
New York, NY 10021
212-744-8205

Marilyn B. Rosanes-Berrett,
   Ph.D.
510 East 89th Street
New York, NY 10128
212-879-0138

Adam Schwartz
179 East 3rd Street, Apt. 23
New York, NY 10009
212-260-7932

NORTH CAROLINA

Dr. Gil Alvarado
230 Landsbury Drive
Durham, NC 27707-2414
919-933-7373

C. J. Wilson, C.N.V.I.
135 Old Bull Creek Road
Marshall, NC 28753
704-689-5740

OHIO

Robert Fridenstine
New Horizons
53166 State Route 681
Reedsville, OH 45772
614-378-6366, 800-755-6360

OREGON

The Joy of Being Center
2400 Siskiyou Boulevard
Ashland, OR 97520
503-482-6579

Anni Azalea
118B Merry Lane
Eugene, OR 97404
503-461-6902

TEXAS

Angelica Jeanne Fitzsimmons,
    C.N.V.I.
3300 Bee Caves Road, Suite 650
Austin, TX 78746
512-327-5683

VERMONT

J. Beth Baldwin
PO Box 1238
Burlington, VT 05402
802-660-2582

VIRGINIA

Lynn Bernard
3500 Royal Palm Arch
Virginia Beach, VA 23452-3707
804-463-2609

WASHINGTON

Beverly Robertson, M.S.
Potential Plus
PO Box 309
Chelan, WA 98816
509-682-4022
509-682-3492

Phyllis Mar
7615-B Aurora Avenue North
Seattle, WA 98103
206-783-8542
206-789-6280

INTERNATIONAL

AUSTRALIA

Luciano Giangiordano
43 Parkview Drive
Ballajura, WA 6066
AUSTRALIA
09-249-1682

Dede Callichy
18 Elovera Terrace
Bray Park 2484
AUSTRALIA
066-72-4748

Tony-Paul Gaynor
62 Aberdeen Road
Busby, NSW 2168
AUSTRALIA
02-607-2125

Wilma Thomson
PO Box 220
Elwood, Melbourne, VIC 3184
AUSTRALIA

Dawn Palm
2 Southgate Court
Kingsley 6026
AUSTRALIA
619-409-1083

Michael Bull
83 William Edward Street
Longueville, NSW 2066
AUSTRALIA
02-418-9271

Janet Goodrich
Natural Vision Improvement
   Teachers Headquarters
Crystal Waters Permaculture
   Village
M.S. 16
Maleny, Queensland 4552
AUSTRALIA
(074) 94 4657
(074) 94 4673 fax

Janet Kenworthy
PO Box 118
Mapleton, QLD 4560
AUSTRALIA
074-457-480

Joan Glengarry
30 Jameson Street
Mosman Park, WA 6012
AUSTRALIA
09-383-3717

Philip McManus
PO Box 1100
Noosa Heads, QLD 4567
AUSTRALIA
074-74-9999

Susanna Wilkerson
PO Box 338
Ravenshoe, QLD 4872
AUSTRALIA
070-970-272

Thelma Kosmina
3 Compton Street
Reservoir, VIC 3073
AUSTRALIA
03-460-2468

Judy Boyd
PO Box 105
Ringwood East, VIC 3135
AUSTRALIA
613-870-8083

Jean Ponchard
2/3 Manion Avenue
Rose Bay, NSW 2029
AUSTRALIA
02-363-2472
02-371-6325

Roslyn Gaye Gowing
108 Main Road
Speer's Point, NSW
AUSTRALIA
049-508-178

Margaret Brady
45 Barrymount Crescent
Toowoomba, QLD 4350
AUSTRALIA
076-326773
076-347725 fax

Deanna Stewart
204 Crystal Brook Road
Wattle Grove, WA 6107
AUSTRALIA
09-453-1111

CANADA

Sachi Nakai
200 Gateway Boulevard,
    Apt. 1517
Don Mills, ONT M3C 1B6
CANADA
416-429-3598

Annemarie Konas
404-345 West 10th Avenue
Vancouver, BC V5Y 1S2
CANADA
604-871-3035

ENGLAND

Pé Lé Hentsch
39 Melton Court, Onslow
    Square
London, SW7
ENGLAND
071-584-9080

Caroline Barrow
Kulu Lodge, Horseleaze Lane
Shipham, Avon BS25 IUQ
ENGLAND
11-44-0934-842297

GERMANY

Christiane Ganser
Furbringerstr. 9, Hh. l. Etage
    Links
10961 Berlin
GERMANY
030-6944497

Gisela Hanschen and Margit
    Kaufman
NVI Teachers
Obentrautstrabe 32,3
10963 Berlin
GERMANY
030-2518501

Uschi Ostermeier-Sitowski
Oberhofer Strasse 28
87471 Durach, Kempten
GERMANY
831-60647

Elke Werkmeister
Tydal 2
D-24852 Eggebek
GERMANY
04609-1561

Ingeborg M. Bücherl
Maistrasse 40
80337 München
GERMANY
089-532-8342

Wolfgang Gillessen
42a Ettalstrasse
81377 München
GERMANY
089-7140814
089-713224

ITALY

Ambretta Rendina
Via Vittoria Colonna 52
20149 Milano
ITALY

NETHERLANDS

Jos Van Rijn
Pr. W. Van Oranjelaan 16
1412 GK Naarden
NETHERLANDS
0-2159-41590

NEW ZEALAND

Tony White
4 Pinetree Lane
Korokoro Petrone, Wellington
NEW ZEALAND
64-4-589-0969

SWITZERLAND

Franz Luethi
Im Buech 9
9247 Henau
SWITZERLAND
073-512270

Endnotes

1. "Don't Worry, You'll Get Used to It!"

1. Ingrid Lorch, "Total Vision," *East West,* April 1990, p. 48.
2. Richard Leviton, *Seven Steps to Better Vision,* p. 5.
3. Hazel Dawkins, Ellis Edelman, and Constantine Forkiotis, *Suddenly Successful: How Behavioral Optometry Helps You Overcome Learning, Health, and Behavior Problems,* p. 116
4. Arnold Gesell, et al., Vision, Its Development in Infant and Child, as quoted in Dawkins, Edelman, and Forkiotis, p. 32.
5. Deepak Chopra, *Quantum Healing,* p. 61.
6. Ibid., p. 58 (emphasis added).
7. From lecture given on March 23, 1991, at the Living Enrichment Center, Portland, Oregon.
8. Ibid.

2. What I Learned in School

1. Richard Leviton, *Seven Steps to Better Vision,* p. 11.
2. James H. Allen, *May's Diseases of the Eye,* 24th ed. (Baltimore: Williams & Wilkins, 1968), p. 295.
3. Raymond L. Gottlieb, "Neuropsychology of Myopia," *Journal of Optometric Vision Development,* vol. 13, no. 1 (March 1982), pp. 3–27.
4. Ibid., p. 8 (emphasis added) and p. 23.
5. Ibid., p. 9.
6. Data from Hazel Dawkins, Ellis Edelman, and Constantine Forkiotis, *Suddenly Successful: How Behavioral Optometry Helps You Overcome Learning, Health, and Behavior Problems,* pp. 84–86.
7. Theodore Grosvenor, "The Results of Myopia Control Studies Have Not Been Encouraging," *Journal of Behavioral Optometry,* vol. 4, no. 1, pp. 17–19.
8. Gottlieb, p. 4.
9. Dawkins, Edelman, and Forkiotis, p. 86.

10. M. J. Hirsch, "The Refraction of Children." In M. J. Hirsch and R. E. Wick, eds., *Vision of Children* (New York: Chilton, 1963).

11. Dawkins, Edelman, and Forkiotis, p. 85.

12. Gottlieb, p. 11.

13· William Bates, *The Cure of Imperfect Sight by Treatment Without Glasses* (New York: Central Fixation Publishing, 1920).

14.· Gottlieb, p. 5.

15. Jennifer Nelson, "Visual Acuity in Myopia." O.D. dissertation, College of Optometry, Pacific University.

16.· Grosvenor.

17. "Decreased Uncorrected Vision After a Period of Distance Fixation with Spectacle Wear," *Optometry and Vision Science,* vol. 70, no. 7, pp. 528–31.

3. An Experiment on the Workings of the Mind

1. Raymond L. Gottlieb, "Neuropsychology of Myopia," *Journal of Optometric Vision Development,* vol. 13, no. 1 (March 1982), p. 15.

2. Marie A. Marrone, "Peripheral Awareness," *Journal of Behavioral Optometry,* vol. 2, no. 1, pp. 7–11.

3. William Bates, *The Bates Method for Better Eyesight Without Glasses,* p. 47.

4. Ibid., p. 47 (emphasis added).

5. Aldous Huxley, *The Art of Seeing,* p. 45.

4. Open Focus: Let Your Vision Escape Your Eyes

1. Aldous Huxley, *The Art of Seeing,* p. 25.

2. Jacques Lusseyran, *And There Was Light,* pp. 16–17.

3. Ibid., pp. 32–33.

4. Larry Dossey, *Recovering the Soul* (New York: Bantam Books, 1989), pp. 18–19.

5. Arthur Zajonc, *Catching the Light: The Entwined History of Light and Mind,* pp. 4–6 (emphasis added).

6. Quoted in ibid., p. 205 (emphasis added).

7. Rupert Sheldrake, *A New Science of Life: The Hypothesis of Formative Causation,* revised and expanded ed. (Los Angeles: Jeremy P. Tarcher, 1981), back cover (emphasis added).

8. Ibid., review from *World Medicine* quoted on back cover.

9. Ibid., p. 250.

10. Raymond L. Gottlieb, "Neuropsychology of Myopia," *Journal of Optometric Vision Development,* vol. 13, no. 1 (March 1982), p. 12.

11. Ibid., pp. 17–18.

12. Lusseyran, p. 17–21.

5. Seeing Through the Fear

1. Raymond L. Gottlieb, "Neuropsychology of Myopia," *Journal of Optometric Vision Development,* vol. 13, no. 1 (March 1982), p. 10.

2. Raymond L. Gottlieb, "Eliminate Myopia? It's Not So Far-fetched," *20/20,* vol. 10, no. 5.

3. Lisette Scholl, *Visionetics: The Holistic Way to Better Eyesight* (Garden City, N.Y.: Doubleday, 1978), p. 22.

4. Gottlieb, "Neuropsychology of Myopia," p. 10.

5. Scholl, pp. 22–23.

6. Gottlieb, "Neuropsychology of Myopia," pp. 4, 11.

7. Ibid., p. 11.

8. "Studies Offer a New Understanding of Myopia," *New York Times,* May 18, 1993.

9. Michael Talbot, *The Holographic Universe,* p. 99.

10. "Alter Personalities Vary in Dominance, EEG, Muscle Tone," *Brain/Mind Bulletin,* December 30, 1985.

11. "Personalities Differ in Visual Systems," *Brain/Mind Bulletin,* October 3, 1983.

12. Talbot, pp. 98–100.

13. "Personalities Differ in Visual Systems," *Brain/Mind Bulletin,* October 3, 1983.

7. Change Your Vision, Change Your Life!

1. Hazel Dawkins, Ellis Edelman, and Constantine Forkiotis, *Suddenly Successful: How Behavioral Optometry Helps You Overcome Learning, Health, and Behavior Problems.*

8. Take Off Your Glasses and See!

1. Bija Bennett, *Breathing into Life* (San Francisco: HarperSanFrancisco, 1993), p. 3.

2. Aldous Huxley, *The Art of Seeing,* p. 54.

3. Ibid., p. 89–90.

4. Darrell Boyd Harmon, *The Coordinated Classroom* (Grand Rapids, Mich.: American Seating Company, 1951).

5. "Vision Training Program Ups IQ, Cuts Rearrest Rate of Juvenile Delinquents," *Brain/Mind Bulletin,* vol. 8 (1983).

11. Living Clearly: Being Present and Staying Current

1. "Writing Your Way to Better Health," *Health Consumer's Health & Wellness Report,* vol. 4, no. 2. (Summary of J. W. Pennebaker, "Putting Stress into Words: Health, Linguistic and Therapeutic Implications," *Behaviour Research and Therapy,* vol. 31 [1993], pp. 539–48.)

2. From lecture given on March 23, 1991, at the Living Enrichment Center, Portland, Oregon.

13. Seeing the Invisible

1. Quoted in Arthur Zajonc, *Catching the Light: The Entwined History of Light and Mind,* p. ix.

2. Ibid., p. 2.

3. George C. Brainard et al., "Ultraviolet Regulation of Neuroendocrine and Circadian Physiology in Rodents and the Visual Evoked Response in Children," in *Biological Responses to UVA Radiation,* ed. Frederick Urbach (Overland Park, Kan.: Valdenmar Publishing Company, 1992).

4. Jack Schwarz, *Human Energy Systems* (New York: E. P. Dutton, 1980), p. 69.

5. Arnold Gesell et al., *Vision, Its Development in Infant and Child,* as quoted in Raymond L. Gottlieb, "Neuropsychology of Myopia," *Journal of Optometric Vision Development,* vol. 13, no. 1 (March 1982), p. 16.

6. Jacques Lusseyran, *And There Was Light,* p. 18.

7. Neville Spearman, *The Boy Who Saw True* (Suffolk, England: Hillman Printers, 1953), pp. 28–29.

8. Ibid., p. 32.

9. Ibid., p. 94.

10. Barbara Ann Brennan, *Hands of Light* (New York: Bantam, 1987), pp. 6–7.

11. Herbert Thurston, *The Physical Phenomena of Mysticism* (Chicago: Henry Regnery Company, 1952).

12. Michael Talbot, *The Holographic Universe,* p. 165.

13. James H. Allen, *May's Diseases of the Eye,* 24th ed. (Baltimore: Williams & Williams, 1968), p. 218.

14. Satprem, *The Mind of the Cells,* trans. Francine Mahak and Luc Venet (New York: Institute for Evolutionary Research, 1989), pp. 89–90.

14. The Truth About Thinking

1. Wendy Marston, "Visual Vignette: Eyes Are Mirrors of the Mind," *Journal of Optometric Vision Development,* vol. 24, no. 1 (Spring 1993), p. 3.

2. William Bates, *The Bates Method for Better Eyesight Without Glasses,* p. 50.

3. Sampooran Singh, "Human Destiny: Integration of Spirituality and Science," *Network: The Scientific and Medical Network Newsletter,* no. 53 (December 1993), pp. 15–17.

4. Ibid.

5. Robert Monroe, *Far Journeys* (New York: Doubleday, 1985), pp. 71–72.

6. Michael Talbot, *The Holographic Universe,* p. 262.

7. Marilyn Ferguson, "Commentary: Crop Circles in a Trackless Field," *Brain/Mind Bulletin,* vol. 18, no. 2 (November 1992).

15. Effortless Seeing, Effortless Learning

1. Valerie Maxwell, "How Lack of Learning Abilities and Vision Functions Lower Self-Esteem," *SOI News,* June 1989.

2. William Ludlam, quoted in ibid., pp. 5–7.

3. Hazel Dawkins, Ellis Edelman, and Constantine Forkiotis, *Suddenly Successful: How Behavioral Optometry Helps You Overcome Learning, Health, and Behavior Problems,* p. 5.

4. In Maxwell, unattributed quote from "developmental optometrists."

5. Mary Meeker, quoted in Maxwell.

6. Dawkins, Edelman, and Forkiotis, p. 15.

7. Maxwell.

8. Dawkins, Edelman, and Forkiotis, p. 141.

9. Maxwell.

10. "Vision Training Provides Window to Brain Change," *Brain/Mind Bulletin,* vol. 7, no. 17.

11. "School Anxiety May Be Major Cause of Myopia," *Brain/Mind Bulletin,* vol. 7, no. 17.

12. Raymond L. Gottlieb, "Neuropsychology of Myopia," *Journal of Optometric Vision Development,* vol. 13, no. 1 (March 1982), p. 9 (emphasis added).

13. "Society May Be Sabotaging Its Own Intelligence," *Brain/Mind Bulletin,* vol. 7, no. 7.

14. "How-To Instructions Inhibit Optimum Performance," *Brain/Mind Bulletin,* vol. 7, no. 17.

15. "Movement Psychology: Freeing 'Postural Beliefs,' " *Brain/Mind Bulletin,* vol. 8, no. 8 (April 18, 1983).

16. "Gelb: Freeing the Body to Free the Mind for Learning," *Brain/Mind Bulletin,* vol. 9, no. 3 (January 2, 1984).

16. How to Learn Without Effort

1. Joseph Chilton Pierce, *Evolution's End: Claiming the Potential of Our Intelligence* (San Francisco: HarperSanFrancisco, 1992), p. 13 (emphasis added).

Epilogue: Open Living

1. David Bohm, "Of Matter and Meaning: The Super-Implicate Order," *ReVision* (Spring 1983).

Bibliography and Further Reading

App, John. *Secrets of Seeing Without Glasses or Contacts.* Self-published, 1990.

Bates, William. *The Bates Method for Better Eyesight Without Glasses.* New York: Henry Holt & Co., 1981.

Benjamin, Harry. *Better Sight Without Glasses.* New York: Thorsons/ HarperCollins, 1984.

Bohm, David, and F. David Peat. *Science, Order, and Creativity: A Dramatic New Look at the Creative Roots of Science and Life.* New York: Bantam, 1987.

Chopra, Deepak. *Quantum Healing.* New York: Bantam, 1989.

Corbett, Margaret Darst. *Help Yourself to Better Sight.* North Hollywood, Calif.: Wilshire Book Co., 1949.

Dawkins, Hazel Richmond, Ellis Edelman, and Constantine Forkiotis. *Suddenly Successful: How Behavioral Optometry Helps You Overcome Learning, Health, and Behavior Problems.* Santa Ana, Calif.: Optometric Extension Program Foundation, 1991

Forrest, Elliot B. *Stress and Vision.* Santa Ana, Calif.: Optometric Extension Program Foundation, 1988.

Friedman, Edward, with Kalia Lilow. *Dr. Friedman's Vision Training Program.* New York: Bantam, 1983.

Goodrich, Janet. *Natural Vision Improvement.* Berkeley: Celestial Arts, 1985.

Huxley, Aldous. *The Art of Seeing.* Berkeley: Creative Arts Book Company, 1982.

Kaplan, Robert-Michael. *Seeing Without Glasses.* Hillsboro, Ore.: Beyond Words Publishing, 1994.

———. *The Power Behind Your Eyes.* Rochester, Vt.: Inner Traditions, 1995.

Kavner, Richard S. *Your Child's Vision: A Parent's Guide to Seeing, Growing, and Developing.* New York: Fireside/Simon & Schuster, 1985.

Kavner, Richard S., and Lorraine Dusky. *Total Vision.* Millwood, N.Y.: Kavner Books, 1978.

Leviton, Richard. *Seven Steps to Better Vision: Easy, Practical and Natural Techniques That Will Improve Your Eyesight.* Brookline, Mass.: EastWest/ Natural Health Books, 1992.

Liberman, Jacob. *Light: Medicine of the Future.* Santa Fe: Bear & Co., 1991.

Lusseyran, Jacques. *And There Was Light.* New York: Parabola Books, 1987.

Markert, Christopher. *Seeing Well Again Without Your Glasses.* C. W. Daniel Co., 1981.

Rosanes-Berrett, Marilyn B. *Do You Really Need Glasses?* Barrytown, N.Y.: Pulse/Station Hill Press, 1990.

Rotté, Joanna, and Koji Yamamoto. *A Holistic Guide to Healing the Eyesight.* Japan Publications, 1986.

Schneider, Meir. *Self-Healing: My Life and Vision.* New York: Arkana/Viking Penguin, 1987.

Seiderman, Arthur S., and Steven E. Marcus. *20/20 Is Not Enough.* New York: Alfred A. Knopf, 1989.

Selby, John. *The Visual Handbook: The Complete Guide to Seeing More Clearly.* Rockport, Mass.: Element Books, 1987.

Talbot, Michael. *The Holographic Universe.* New York: HarperCollins, 1991.

Zajonc, Arthur. *Catching the Light: The Entwined History of Light and Mind.* New York: Bantam, 1993.

To contact Jacob Liberman, or to request a free newsletter with information about his workshop and lecture schedule, please write to:

Universal Light Technology (ULT)
PO Box 520
Carbondale, CO 81623

. . . or call ULT at:
800-81-LIGHT (800-815-4448)
303-927-0100
303-927-0101 fax

Index

About the Author

Dr. Jacob Liberman holds a Doctorate in Optometry (O.D.) from the Southern College of Optometry and a Ph.D. in Vision Science for his pioneering work in phototherapy. Formerly president of the College of Syntonic Optometry, Dr. Liberman is now president of Universal Light Technology, Ltd., an Aspen, Colorado, business doing research, development, and educational seminars on phototherapy and phototherapeutic devices. Since 1973, Dr. Liberman has used his methods effectively with more than thirty thousand patients and, through his extensive lecture and seminar schedule, he has shared his discoveries with thousands of audiences throughout the world. Dr. Jacob Liberman is a pioneer in the therapeutic use of light and color and their relationship to human consciousness and personal transformation. His first book, *Light: Medicine of the Future* (Santa Fe: Bear & Co., 1991), is considered to be on the cutting edge of enlightened technology.